KIA KAHA,
KIA MANA.

# Earthrace

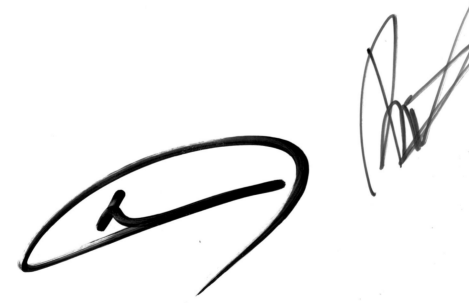

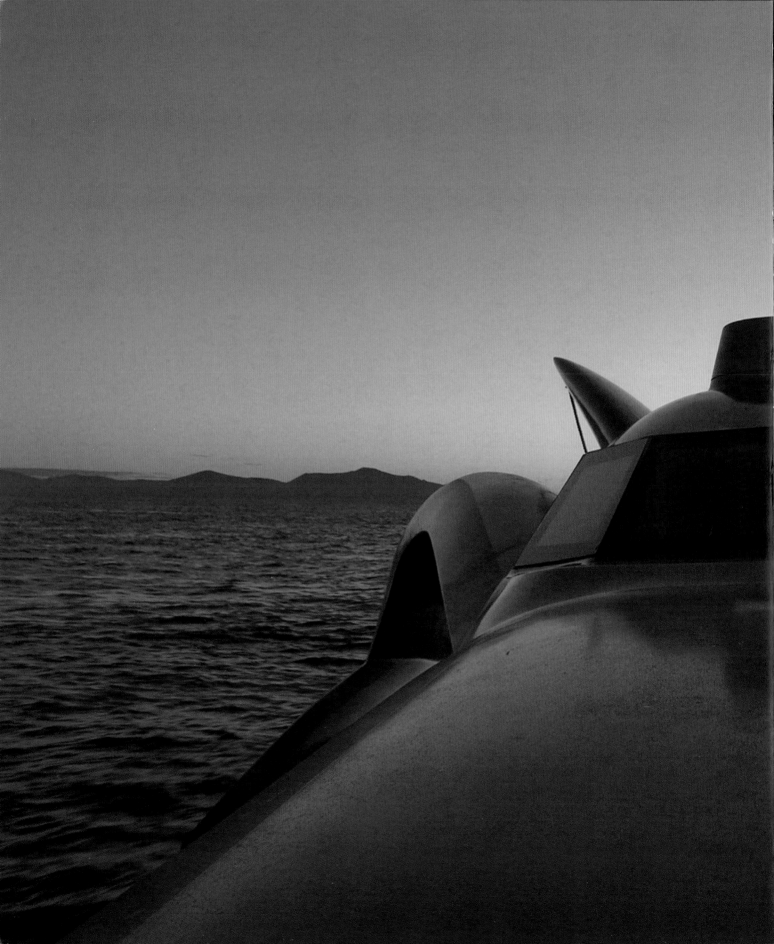

# Earthrace

## Futuristic Adventures on the High Seas

Pete Bethune

Hodder Moa

**National Library of New Zealand Cataloguing-in-Publication Data**

Bethune, Pete.

Earthrace : futuristic adventures on the high seas / by

Pete Bethune.

ISBN 978-1-86971-124-5

1. Bethune, Pete—Travel. 2. Earthrace (Trimaran)

3. Adventure and adventurers—New Zealand—Biography

4. Voyages around the world.

797.1250993—dc 22

A Hodder Moa Book

Published in 2008 by Hachette Livre NZ Ltd

4 Whetu Place, Mairangi Bay

Auckland, New Zealand

Designed and produced by Hachette Livre NZ Ltd

Printed by SNP Leefung Printers Limited, China

Front and back cover photographs: Earthrace

# Contents

This book is dedicated to the most amazing three people in my life: my stunning wife Sharyn, and my two wonderful daughters Danielle and Alycia.

# Earthrace legends

The backbone of Earthrace has been an army of volunteers who have selflessly dedicated days, weeks and in some cases years of their lives to make this project happen. Towards the end of Earthrace I started calling these people legends, because that's what they are, although their contributions were seldom recognised. They just kept turning up day after day, city after city and country after country, with no reward other than perhaps the thought that they can contribute. Below are the legends that came to mind in writing this book. There are many others and my apologies for those of you whom I've missed. The team and I are eternally grateful to you all.

Steve Adams — Auckland, NZ
Sven Aerts — Belgium
Ken Alchin — Auckland, NZ
Riaan Alers — Cape Town, South Africa
John Allen — Matamata, NZ
Carlos Baez — San Juan, Puerto Rico
Mathew Besler — Chicago, IL, USA
Rid Bestwick — Vancouver, Canada
Bazza Bethune — Riverton, NZ
Sharyn Bethune — Auckland, NZ
Danielle Bethune — Auckland, NZ
Alycia Bethune — Auckland, NZ
Graham Bethune — Auckland, NZ
Mark Blackham — Wellington, NZ
Bruce Blackwell — Mississippi, USA
Michelle Bond-Ewart — Hamilton, NZ
Alain Brideson (Buddha) — Auckland, NZ
Deni Brideson — Auckland, NZ
Gregg Brideson — Auckland, NZ
Toby Brocklehurst — Panama City, Panama
Tom Brooks — Opotiki, NZ
Peter Brown — San Jose, CA, USA
Harvey Brunt — Auckland, NZ
Jim Burkett — Tampa, FL, USA
Matthew Butler — Houston, TX, USA
John Carroll — Portland, OR, USA
James Cato — Auckland, NZ

Commandante Castro — Puerto Quetzal, Guatemala
Leo Chan — Baltimore, MD, USA
Sheila Chandor, San Francisco, CA, USA
Ryan Christiansen — San Juan, Puerto Rico
Andy Christman — San Diego, CA, USA
Martin Conway — UK
Chris Coppin — Gisborne, NZ
Tim Costar — Auckland, NZ
Ron Crafts — Utah, USA
Nigel Cusans — Panama City, Panama
Paul Debenham — Tauranga, NZ
Jill DeFelice — Delaware, USA
Anthony Destifano — Wilmington, NC, USA
Jules Dorian — Melbourne, Australia
Adrian Erange — Cork, Ireland
Paul Ewart — Hamilton, NZ
Paul Farrington — Bermuda
Andrew Ferguson — Auckland, NZ
Kate Folchert — Seattle, USA
Scott Fratcher — USA
Jefferey Fredenburgh — Bridgetown, Barbados
Liza Fredenburgh — Bridgetown, Barbados
Terry Froggly — Auckland, NZ
Vikki Galloway — Mexico City, Mexico
Jeff Gibbs — Fort Lauderdale, FL, USA
Carlos Gonzalez — San Juan, Puerto Rico

Joe Grabill — South Bend, IN, USA
Keren Harris — Wellington, NZ
Richard Hemphill — San Juan, Puerto Rico
Claire Hardin — Panama City, Panama
KC Hardin — Panama City, Panama
Glen Harvey — Nelson, NZ
Keith Herbert — Vancouver, BC, Canada
Len Herchen — Calgary, Canada
Ove Herlogsen — Gothenburg, Sweden
Willie Hetaraka — Te Kauwhata, NZ
Ryan Heron — Wanganui, NZ
Jenna Higgins — Jefferson City, MO, USA
Harry and Penelope Hill — San Diego, CA, USA
Jason Hoar — San Luis Obispo, CA, USA
Chad Hock, Wilmington, SC, USA
Matthew Houptman — Auckland, NZ
Kerry Hourigan — New York, NY, USA
Penelope Hill — San Diego, CA, USA
Dima Ivanov — Auckland, NZ
Bobbo Jetmundsen — Atlanta, GA, USA
Joe Jobe — Jefferson City, MO, USA
Rob Jones — Vancouver, BC, Canada
Tony Jordan — Vancouver, BC, Canada
Sean Kelly — Whangamata, NZ
Ryan Kiefer — Nebraska, USA
John King — Auckland, NZ

Kelly and Bob King — Maui, HA, USA
Jennifer Koseklin (Bud chick) — Koror, Palau
Harold Kraus — Kansas, MO, USA
Barbara Kriz — Opua, NZ
Tina Kula — Maalaia, HI, USA
Mark Kupsko — Chicago, IL, USA
Jennifer Kuntz — Destin, FL, USA
Adrian Lake — Newcastle, Australia
Scott Lengell — Boston, MA, USA
Peter Maire — Auckland, NZ
Marcel Manders — Auckland, NZ
Jose J Marti — San Juan, Puerto Rico
Tracy Martin — Hamilton, NZ
Mike Matthews — UK
Molly McCrackin, San Diego, CA, USA
John (Cadillac) McDaniel — Miami, FL, USA
Bob McDavitt — Auckland, NZ
Jeff McDermott — Charleston, SC, USA
Geoff McGlashan — Nelson, NZ
Sheryl McGlashan — Nelson, NZ
Brian Mead — Auckland, NZ
Graeme Mead — Hamilton, NZ
Marty Mead — Orcas Islands, WA, USA
Ravvi Mikkelsen — Seattle, WA
Jeff McDermott — Charleston, SC, USA
Patrick Madden — Majuro, Marshall Islands
Paul McAlister, New York, NY, USA
Tom McNicholl — Auckland, NZ
Marty Mead — Orcas Islands, WA, USA
Pete Milborn — Maui, HI, USA
Mal Molgard — Boston, MA, USA
Meghan Murphy — San Francisco, CA, USA
Elio Muller — Tampa, FL, USA
Tim Murray — Cessnock, NSW, Australia
Dave and Sharon Nelson — Hilton Head, SC, USA
Norman — Bridgetown, Barbados
Je Nowak — Auckland, NZ
Donita O'Dell — Alaska, USA
Fei Fei Ong — Singapore
Elizabeth Paradiso — Maui, HI, USA
Hedley Pearce — Dunedin, NZ
Marta Perez — NY, USA
David Perez — NY, USA
Edgar Perez — San Francisco, CA, USA
Chris Peterson — Los Angeles, CA, USA
Wade Peyer — Mobile, AL, USA
Pit, Flash and Jason — Philadelphia, USA
John Plaza — Seattle, USA
Florian Prem — Germany
Hemi Rau — Hopuhopu, NZ
Naren Raju — Singapore
Martin Rees — Auckland, NZ
Megan Reeves — Auckland, NZ
Wayne Renner — Tauranga, NZ
Carl Revine — St Petersburg, FL, USA
Ngapera Riley — New York, NY, USA
George Ritchie — Christchurch, NZ
Jesse Rhodes — Charleston, SC, USA
Roberto Rush — Panama City, Panama
Jake Roy — Charleston, SC, USA
Grant Saar — Vancouver, Canada

Ian Sanchez — Charleston, SC, USA
Torsten Sandmark — Dunedin, NZ
Michael Sarin — Phoenix, AZ, USA
Mat Sarin — San Diego, CA, USA
Rae Sarin — San Diego, CA, USA
Kiera Schwarz — Kemah, TX, USA
Guy Sheetz — Charleston, SC, USA
John Sheetz — San Diego, CA, USA
Mike Schimann — Ontario, Canada
Emanual Siedner — Guatemala City, Guatemala
Bruce Sharpe — Bermuda
Matt Stein, Portland, OR, USA
Mich Stein — Portland, OR, USA
Pete Stevens — Panama City, Panama
Martin Stroud — Auckland, NZ
Matt Stott — Auckland, NZ
Sean Sullivan — Houston, TX, USA
Peter Syred — Auckland, NZ
Inia Taylor — Auckland, NZ
Vivien Teo — Singapore
Allison Thompson — USA
Charlene Tighe — Ft Lauderdale, FL, USA
Glen Tindall — Sydney, Australia
Kylie Travers — Auckland, NZ
Peter Trezise — Auckland, NZ
Tom Verry — Jefferson City, MO, USA
Brian Van Buskirk — Portland, OR, USA
Heidi van Buskirk, Portland, OR, USA
Robert van Gool — San Francisco, CA, USA
Randall von Wedel — San Francisco, CA, USA
Colin Walker — UK
Jean Weaver — Wisconsin, USA
Peggy West Stap (the Pegster) — Monterey, CA, USA
Tom Widdle — Portland, OR, USA
Steve Wilkinson — Auckland, NZ
John Williams — Seattle, USA
Ayla Witehira — Whangarei, NZ
Barry Woolsey — Auckland, NZ
Lance Wordsworth — Auckland, NZ
Nicky Wright — Auckland, NZ
Emad Yacoub — Melbourne, Australia
Devann Yata — Oceanside, CA, USA
Roy Yen — Vancouver, Canada
Rob Yoeman — Auckland, NZ
Elise Zevitz — Wisconsin, USA

## Presenting sponsors

Bacassa
Biodiesel Oils NZ Ltd
Calibre Boats
Ciclon
Craig Loomes Design Group
Cummins Mercruiser Diesel
Diab
Germanische Lloyd
Ocean Oasis Panama
South Canterbury Finance
Streetsmart
ZF Marine

## Supporting sponsors

3D Disaster Services — Funding — USA
3M — Signwriting Materials — NZ
Agri Source Fuels — Biodiesel — USA
Agrifuels — Biodiesel — USA
Aladin Travel — Accommodation — Oman
Albany Chartered Accountants — Accounting — NZ
Alphatron — Inverter — NZ
Amcor Packaging — Plastic Film — NZ
Ameron Coating — Coatings — NZ
Ashmar — Construction Consumables — NZ
Assist America — 24hr Medical Assistance — USA
Aurora Marine — Wax Coating — USA
Auckland Plastic Surgery — Liposuction — NZ
Autex — Marine Carpets — NZ
Banjo — Valves — USA
Banyantree — Funding — Barbados
Baytex — Marquee — NZ
Better Biodiesel — Funding — USA
Bioenergy Plantations — Biodiesel — USA
Biodiesel & Fuels De Puerto Rico — Biodiesel — Puerto Rico
Biox Corporation — Biodiesel — USA
BP — Fuel — NZ
Brendon Engineering — Engineering — NZ
C Map — Electronic Charts — United Kingdom
Campa Iberia — Biodiesel — Spain
CamSensor Technologies — Various — NZ
Capital Instruments — Gauges — NZ
Carotech — Biodiesel — Singapore
Century Batteries — 12V Batteries — NZ
Clean Green Car Company — Car — NZ
Coast Long Beach Hotel — Accommodation — USA
Coastguard — Crew Training — NZ
Codescan — Funding — NZ
Columbia Sportswear — Clothing — USA
Corporate Water Brands — Bottled Water — NZ
Crystal Flash Energy — Funding — USA
Daestra — Online Location Tracking — NZ
Deckgrip — Marine Antislip — NZ
Delfino Maritime Agency — Canal Crossing — Panama
Delta Fuels — Biodiesel — USA
Detyens Shipyard — Refit — Charleston, SC, USA
Diogene Marine — Prototype Engine — Mauritius
Dogcam Sport UK — Pencil Cameras — UK
Donaghys — Ropes — NZ
Dometic — Blackwater Tank — USA
Domex — Sleeping Bags — NZ
Driscoll Boatworks — Dock Facilities — USA
DPS — Online Sales — NZ
Earth Biofuels — Funding — USA
ECO 5 — Underwater Coating — USA
EECA — Funding — NZ
Elvex — Headphones — USA
Endeavour Express — Film Boat — NZ
Engel — 12 Fridge — South Africa

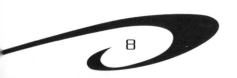

Engineering Plastics — O-Rings — NZ
ESI — Fuel System Design — USA
Euro Inflatables — Fenders — NZ
European Biodiesel Board — Funding — Belgium
Farallon Electronics — Data Communications — USA
Fletcher Aluminium — Aluminium — NZ
FLIR — Infra Red Night Vision — USA
Fortrec — Biodiesel — Singapore
Fortress Anchors — Anchor — USA
Fortune Manning — Legal Counsel — NZ
Fosters — Cleats — NZ
Fuman Graphics — Graphics — NZ
Gear Locker — Clothing — NZ
General Marine Services — Various — NZ
Glidecam — Camera Stabiliser — USA
Go Deep Sea — Offshore Filming — NZ
Greenmount Manufacturing — CNC Machining — NZ
Green Marine — Photography — NZ
Hallmark Marine — Driveshaft Machining — Australia
Harbour Yachts — Prototype — NZ
HCD — Fluid Connectors — NZ
Heletranz — Aerial Filming — NZ
Hella Marine — Lights — NZ
Helly Hansen — Clothing — NZ
Henderson Rental Cars — Truck — NZ
Herman Pacific — Timber — NZ
High Modulus — Composite Materials — NZ
Hirepool — Various — NZ
HJ Cooper — Copper — NZ
Hobecca — Hand Tools — NZ
Huhtamaki — Paper Plates — NZ
Hydroflow — Hosing — NZ
Icom — SSB Radio — USA
Idle Arts — Media Player — NZ
IFM Efector — Sensors — NZ
Imagepac — Digital Printing — NZ
Imperium Renewables — Race Fuel — USA
Imtra — Windscreen Washers — USA
Indian River Marina — Biodiesel — USA
International Machine Group — Various — NZ
ITM — Timber — NZ
ITT Industries — Pumps — USA
Jeppersen — PC Navigation System — USA
Kata — Camera Packs — USA
Kilwell — Carbon Tubes — NZ
Koken Tools — Socket Set — NZ
Konings — Graphics — NZ
Laminex — MDF — NZ
Lewmar — Snatch Block — UK
Lion Breweries — Beer (heaps of it) — NZ
Loop — Music — NZ
Lulus Homeport — Accommodation — India
Lusty & Blundell — Various — NZ
M>Post — Multimedia — NZ
Macduff — Chain — NZ
Maddrens — Timber — NZ
Mag & Turbo Warehouse — Steering Wheel — NZ
Majestic Entertainment — Stereo — Australia

Marathon Products — Bilge Kleen — NZ
Marine Industry Association — Network — NZ
Mark Tours — Accommodation — Egypt
Massey High School — Students — NZ
Matrix Computing — Finite Element Analysis — NZ
Maxwell Marine — Hatches, Winch — NZ
Mencast — Propeller Maintenance — USA
Merle Tex — Possum Fur Socks — NZ
MetService — Weather Forecasting — NZ
Mico Metals — Aluminium — NZ
Moko Ink — Maori Graphics — NZ
Moretti Yachts — Funding — St Petersburg, FL, USA
Mr Binz — Waste Removal — NZ
Multistrut — Cable Trunking — NZ
Mums Original — Food Supplements — USA
National Biodiesel Board — Funding — Jefferson City, MI, USA
Navman — Electronics — NZ
Neco Marine — Docking — Palau
Netactive — Website — NZ
New Zealand Couriers — Courier — NZ
New Zealand Crane Hire — Cranes — NZ
New Zealand Police — Youth Development — NZ
North Sails — Pipe Cots — NZ
North Shore Canvas — Canvas — NZ
North Shore Laser Cutters — Laser Cutters — NZ
Nomen — Cleats — Germany
Norcross — Printing — NZ
Northstar — Radar — USA
NZ Marine.com — Marine Network — NZ
One Degree 15 Marina — Various — Singapore
Operation Corporate Training — Emergency Gear — USA
Oakley — Sunglasses — USA
Orano — Orange Juice — NZ
Orca — Wetsuits — NZ
Orcon — Website Hosting — NZ
Pacific Biodiesel — Biodiesel — Hawaii
Palmetto Biofuels — Biodiesel — USA
Parker Hannifin — Hydraulics — NZ
Permark — Labels — NZ
Phonak — Communications Systems — NZ
Pilkington Glass — Windscreen — NZ
Pizza Hut — Pizza — NZ
Plavan Fuels — Biodiesel — USA
Port St Charles — Marina — Barbados
Portastore Containers — Container — NZ
Powerflow — Exhaust — NZ
Primus — Biodiesel Cooker — Sweden
Profusion — Funding — USA
Pyrotech — Fireworks — NZ
RAL — Marine Service — Spain
R&R Sport — Wakeboard — NZ
Racepro — Bucket Seats — NZ
Racor — Fuel Filters — USA
Rescue Tape — Tape — USA
Rex Castors — Wheels — NZ

Ritchie — Compass — USA
RLA Polymers — PVA — NZ
Rocket Signtists — Signwriting — NZ
Rule — Bilge Pumps — USA
Safety At Sea — Safety Equipment — NZ
Sail NZ — Docking — NZ
Sandvik — Driveshafts — NZ
Sam's Tours — Wicked Day Out — Palau
Seagate — Data Storage — USA
Security Assesments.com — Funding — USA
Senate Communications — PR Counsel — NZ
Serada — Stainless BBQ — NZ
Servotech — Temperature Sensors — NZ
Sheetz Motorsports — Funding — USA
Sick — Sensors — NZ
Sika — Sealants — NZ
Skanska — Funding — Puerto Rico
Skymate — Satellite Communications — USA
Sol Atlantic — Biodiesel — USA
Sonoco Packaging — Packaging — NZ
Sopac — Hatches — NZ
Soy Power Biodiesel — Biodiesel — USA
Specialised Communications — Video Production Equipment — USA
Stonecroft Wines — Wine — NZ
Stormcase — Protective Cases — USA
Styrobeck Plastics — Polystyrene — NZ
System Controls — Electrical Design — NZ
Tecma — Carbon Toilet — Italy
TE Hudgins — Centrifuge — USA
Tenob Marine — Various — NZ
Terry Frogley Design — Graphics — NZ
Time Xtender — Funding — USA
Tides Marine — Shaft Seals — USA
TMQ — Steering System — Australia
Toshiba — Laptops — NZ
Trident Marine Systems — Exhaust Hose — USA
Trinity Hills Wines — Wine — NZ
Unitec — Multimedia — NZ
University of Waikato — Composite Development — NZ
Viking — Liferafts — Denmark
Villas la Lupita — Accommodation — Guatemala
Vulkan — Couplings — Australia
Waikato Motor Group — Car — NZ
Water Wizards — Ocean Photography — USA
West Coast Reduction — Funding — Canada
West Marine — Various — USA
Wild South — Wines — NZ
World Power — Electrical Installation — NZ
World Prep — Emergency Grab Bag — USA
Wright Communications — Media Counsel — NZ
X-Cats — Stickers — United Kingdom
Yacht Lifeline — Medic Training — NZ
Zenergy — Biodiesel — USA

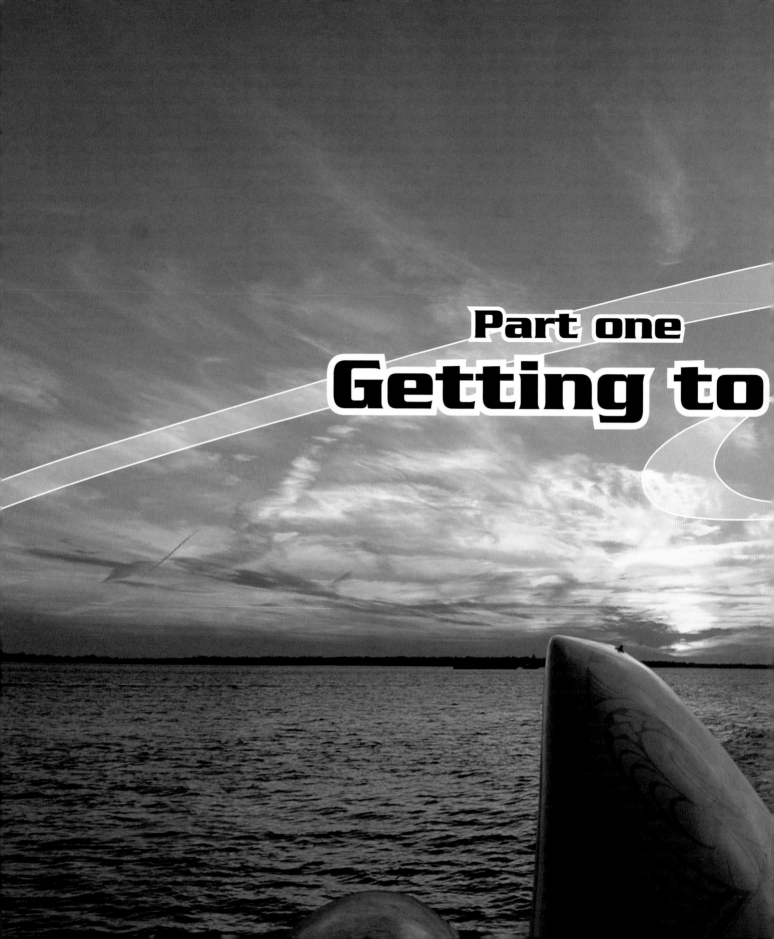

# Part one
# Getting to

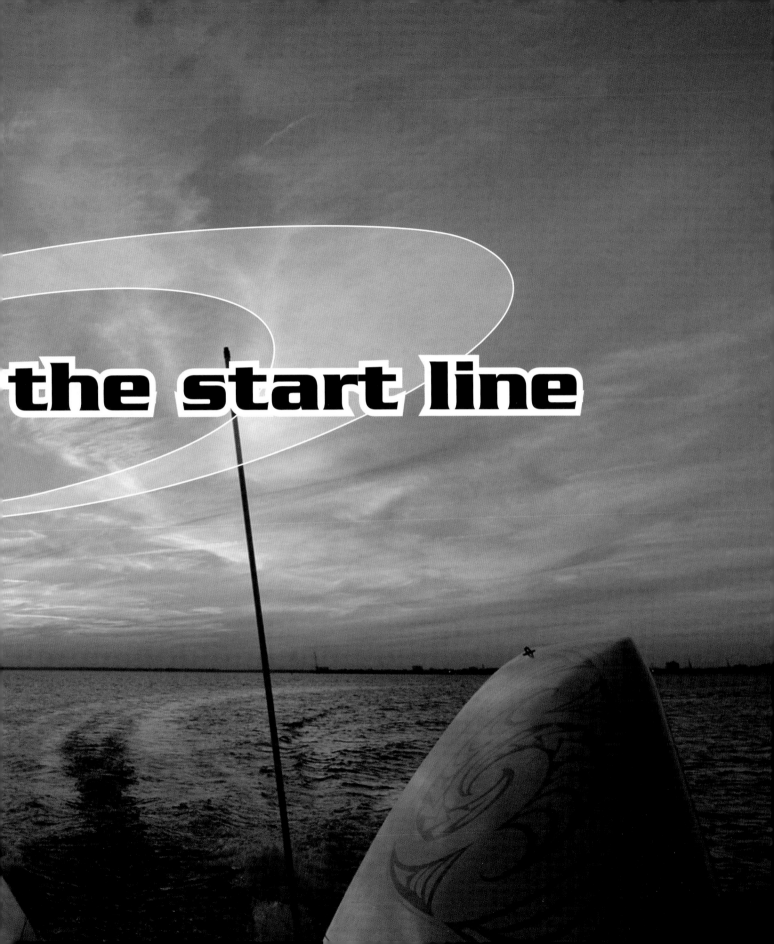

# the start line

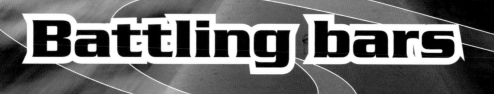

# Battling bars

'That sea looks nasty. You sure you still want to go out?' The gravelly voice coming in over our VHF sounds worried. Local Coastguard have escorted us out to the notorious Raglan bar, and what stands there to greet us, some 400 metres away, are some of the biggest waves I've ever seen. Even where we are, well back from the shallow areas of sand that have the waves standing up and crashing down, the surge and swell are constant and intimidating. 'We'll be fine,' I reply nervously over the VHF, as I push forward on the two throttles of *Earthrace*.

Our speed ramps up and suddenly we're past the Coastguard vessel, which has wisely decided not to make the crossing, and heading for the first big wall of water.

It hits us directly on the bow, a five-metre wave of rolling white water, slowing us down by several knots and sending a shudder down the carbon frame of *Earthrace*. The windscreen is covered in white water and the cabin goes dark as we're engulfed. Seconds later and the bow dips down as we emerge out the other side, the windscreen revealing the next monster only a few seconds away.

The next wave takes longer to clear, leaving us just a split second of vision before the following wave is on us. Then our vision is gone completely, as several waves in a row tear over us, white water now seemingly permanently covering our windscreen. I can feel our bearing has shifted to starboard, the last wave smashing into our port-side bow and pushing us off course.

## 'We need to steer 190 degrees!' I yell at the three crew huddled in the helm beside me

I glance down at our GPS, checking our track, but it's struggling to keep up with the constant changes in direction. Another wave comes crashing down, sending us further to starboard, and pushing us closer to trouble on the sand banks. 'Check the old course,' I say to myself, glancing down at the GPS. A clear map image lights up for a few seconds, just long enough for me to see our old course into Raglan Harbour some three days earlier.

'We need to steer 190 degrees!' I yell at the three crew huddled in the helm beside me.

There's a pregnant pause with none of them saying anything. 'Check the compass and give me the direction!' I yell again, suddenly acutely aware I've got three inexperienced crew with me. I steal a look at the compass: 230 degrees. Well off course. Four turns of the wheel and we're on full lock to port, but each time we start to turn, another wave sends us back to around 230. I push the starboard throttle further forward and ease off on the port, something I know will assist. Over a sequence of five or six waves we gradually swing back to 190. I take it further to 180 to bring us back away from the sand banks that I know must be treacherously close to us by now.

White water continues to obscure the windscreen as wave upon wave toss us around. Suddenly, there's a discernible change in motion, as the bow drops down further and further, and then, amazingly, the windscreen just goes blue. We are going through a large wave, and it's not white water we're engulfed in, but a full, breaking wave. *Earthrace*, as she's designed to do, is submarining — piercing — through the wave. There are bits of weed and flotsam through the water, and the trailing edge of the wave, four or five metres away, is lit up with light dancing off the bubbles and froth on its back face. The boat shudders and groans under the immense energy being transferred through it, and we're jolted around as the wave bursts past. As the trailing edge rolls by, the windscreen miraculously opens up with a clear view of the next big breaking wave, racing towards us.

'Oh my God!' yells Ayla, with genuine fear in her voice. Ayla is a young Maori girl we met in Whangarei a few months earlier, and she has crewed aboard *Earthrace* almost right around New Zealand. I glance over at her and she's staring in horror at the enormous wave arcing down on us.

## 'Hey Pete,' Troffy says with some urgency, 'where do I go to be sick?'

'Man it's an angry sea out here,' I reply, trying not to sound worried, but inside I'm crapping myself.

Each wave, it seems, is a mission. We battle our way through, sometimes falling down into the wave trough behind, then line up for the next monster. By now the waves are approaching seven metres in height but, thankfully, fewer and fewer of them are breaking, and we've gradually eased away from the dangerous bar, littered, I'm all too aware, with old shipwrecks.

'Hey Pete,' Troffy says with some urgency, 'where do I go to be sick?'

I look over at the poor lad who joined us for a three-day trip, anticipating flat water and a spot of fishing, and who's now in one of the worst storms to hit this coast in many years. His face is pale and sickly, and he's clinging to the navigator's seat, seemingly exhausted.

'Not outside,' I yell over the roar of the wind and waves, 'you'll get washed overboard. Just do it in the head.' The head isn't working, but at least the bowl will hold some of it, I think. And it gets the smell away from the rest of us. Troffy staggers back into the galley, clings to the two handles, and starts to convulse. His head and neck move in an 'S' motion as he struggles to contain the vomit erupting inside him. Suddenly, he raises his hand over his mouth to try to stop the inevitable gush of chunder that comes rushing through his fingers, squirting all over the spars and galley floor. Another big wave jolts us sideways, and Troffy collapses onto the floor, his left hand still clinging to the handle. He looks back at us with resignation and defeat in his eyes, and his own vomit swirling around him on the floor.

The stench works its way forward, and there's a slight expansion in my stomach as the first few pangs of seasickness start to work on me. Trevor, who like Troffy is on his first trip aboard *Earthrace*, suddenly scampers back, disappearing into the head. We don't hear him being sick, but there are the telltale splatters of chewed food down his woollen jumper as he emerges a few minutes later. His face is pale, and there's that same look of resignation as he sits down behind Troffy, bracing himself between the two spars, and closing his eyes.

As the day wears on, we gradually work our way northwards towards Auckland. The storm we're in has been brewing offshore for days, and is now honing in on the west coast of New Zealand, centred out from Auckland. 'It'll be an ideal chance to test *Earthrace* in some rough conditions,' I'd said confidently to the team a few days earlier, conscious I'd rather test her here in such conditions than in the middle of the Pacific. It was the end of the tour, though, and most of the crew had scarpered back to Auckland for some rest . . . and now that I'm in the storm, it seems like a foolhardy decision, especially with the current crew's lack of experience. I look back into the galley. Both Troffy and Trevor remain seasick, their only action being continued dry retching and the odd groan.

The steering has gradually become heavier and heavier through the day. 'Pete, I just can't steer this any more,' Ayla finally says to me on dusk. 'The wheel is just too hard to turn, and I keep getting side on to waves.' I climb up into the driver's seat and resume the task of driving us northwards. What I'd do for an autopilot right now, I think. In fact the autopilot is all installed, except for the final wiring. It's one of those jobs lined up for our final refit before leaving New Zealand. But the waves seem manageable. By now we're 30 miles offshore and making progress northwards at around 15 knots.

Then, at around 9pm, the conditions suddenly change. There's a discernible increase in wind, with gusts now howling around us. The waves, which until now had been consistently from the west, also start coming at us from a more northerly direction. We're taking some on the bow and some on our port side, and every now and then a couple combine right in front of us. It's like a giant washing machine, the swirling turbulence tossing us around like a toy. Where before the motion was consistent, it's now changing all the time as different waves come in and smack us.

'Are we OK in these conditions?' Ayla finally says to me. 'These waves are getting really scary.' She's sitting in the navigator's seat nervously clinging to the armrests. *Earthrace* has supposedly been designed for handling big seas. I look out at the huge waves churning past us. Some of them must be at least 12 metres in height, and perhaps the odd larger one.

'I reckon we're sweet, as long as we keep well offshore where there are no reefs or shallows.' Just then an enormous wave starts picking us up from the side. It seems to take ages, as we traverse along its side, and then we're

## Some of these waves are really gnarly

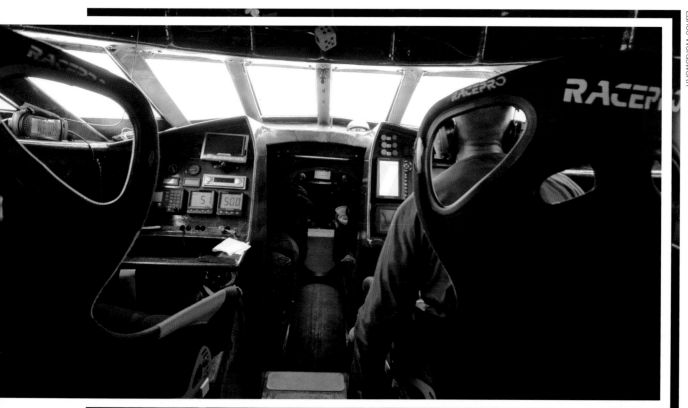

Lance Wordsworth

The *Earthrace* helm feels more like a race car than a boat.

nearly at the top when the crest suddenly gives us a flip, tossing the port sponson (outrigger) up in the air. In an instant it feels like we're going to be tossed right over. Ayla yelps in fear, and our tools and food are sent crashing down on Troffy and Trevor, both now lying on the floor. The sponson finally drops back down as we descend the back of the wave.

'This is madness Pete, we need to go in,' Ayla pleads.

I look down at the GPS. We're about 150 miles from Cape Reinga on the northern tip of New Zealand. It'd take us around 10 hours to get up there I figure, but once around the tip it'd be flat. Another 10 hours of this, though, especially with no one else capable of driving, isn't a pleasant thought. Manukau Harbour lies just 30 miles east of where we are, but I know the bar is extremely dangerous. I grab the VHF and call the Manukau Coastguard.

'As I see it,' I explain to them, 'we have two options. We can continue our voyage north, which will have us around the cape sometime tomorrow morning. Or we can come in over the Manukau bar tonight, and hang out there till the weather clears, although I've never been over the Manukau bar before.'

There's silence on the other end for a few moments, before a broken reply comes through.

'Let me see if we can organise a vessel to escort you over. Stand by.' His voice sounds confident and reassuring despite the marginal reception.

In what seems like an eternity later, we're informed a vessel can meet us outside the harbour to guide us in.

'Are you sure you know how bad these conditions are out here?' I ask the operator. 'Some of these waves are really gnarly.'

'Yes, we're well aware of the conditions,' is his reply. 'The storm has cut power to half of Auckland, and I expect it's rather unpleasant out there now.'

We head in to the coordinates the Coastguard gives us and wait, with our bow pointing into the waves. Eventually, the radio squawks. '*Earthrace, Earthrace*, this is *Rescue 1*.' Man, how good it is to hear his voice. He explains they have seen us directly west of them, and we're given instructions to head east until we come in astern of them.

By now, Troffy has recovered enough to help. He stands in the helm looking for *Rescue 1*, which is somewhere ahead of us among the massive waves. 'Is that them there?' he says enthusiastically, pointing at a solid white light off in the distance. It seems like a long way off, and like a moth to a light, we start heading towards it. I'm scanning the radar for any sign of a blip, but nothing shows. Several miles later and it feels we're still no closer to the light at all. Are they moving ahead at the same speed as us I wonder?

Troffy and I are starting to have doubts about the light being from a boat at all, so we stop, just as *Rescue 1* comes back on the VHF, asking for our coordinates. I'm reading them out when a wave starts to pick us up beam on. As we roll up the wave, we tilt further and further, until I'm standing on the wall, still hanging desperately onto the steering wheel — and a split second later I've got one foot on the roof and one on the wall. We're flipping over, and my worst nightmare is about to come true, as the massive breaking wave carries us along, almost upside down.

Everything not bolted down, including two scaffold planks in the galley, becomes a missile. Maps, phones, food, tools, lights, bolts, engine parts, they all get thrown through the helm, galley and sleeping quarters, although right now it seems the least of our worries. It actually feels like the breaking wave is carrying us along, then, somehow — and I still don't know why or how — the boat flipped back upright. The starboard spar shudders as its sponson digs into the wave, and we all collapse in a heap on the floor. For a few more seconds, though, it seems we're safe.

I throw *Earthrace* back in gear and am surprised when she leaps forward, both engines having survived the violence. We turn back out to sea, now heading directly into the massive waves, while the Coastguard repeatedly calls us. Finally, I get back on the VHF, the Coastguard relieved, I'm sure, to hear we're still intact.

We're given a new set of coordinates where *Rescue 1* is waiting for us, but on entering them in our GPS, it shows them around Kaipara Harbour, some 30 miles north. I enter the coordinates a second time and cannot even see where the point lies. I'm so exhausted and mentally fatigued that simply entering in the numbers correctly is a difficult task. 'Rescue 1, can you please give us a bearing and distance to head for please?' I request over the VHF. Half an hour later and we see them at last, a blue flashing light suddenly appearing for a split second ahead of us.

'Man, am I glad to see them,' says Troffy, obvious relief in his voice. The feeling of isolation evaporates as we line up behind *Rescue 1*, and head for the notorious bar.

We go directly towards the rocks, a mile or so south of the harbour entrance, while *Rescue 1* keeps giving reassuring instructions.

'We'll be heading in on a bearing of 85 degrees.

Keep nice and close here as the channel narrows.

Just ahead we'll be turning sharply to port.'

This last one comes as a relief, as we're only a hundred or so metres from the rocks when the turn is made, our passage now parallel with the shoreline, which seems dangerously close to our starboard side.

On making the turn, we also find ourselves suddenly close to *Rescue 1* and looking in on their stern. 'Oh my God, look how small they are,' says Ayla in amazement. What they're in is a little nine-metre Naiad rigid inflatable. Great boats, but in these conditions it's amazing they even made it over the bar at all, I think. It feels bad enough in a 24-metre vessel, let alone being in that little thing.

# We're close enough to see two people clinging to the aluminium frame as the boat reaches tipping point

Suddenly, they turn to port, pointing their bow out to sea, and an enormous wall of water picks them up. They're vertical on the wall and being driven back towards the rocks, seemingly totally at the wave's mercy. We're close enough to see two people clinging to the aluminium frame as the boat reaches tipping point.

*Rescue 1* somehow grinds her way to the top of the wave, and then races down the back face, towards the second monster now bearing down on them. They scale this one, turn to starboard, and put the hammer down, hurtling towards the safety of the harbour. It's the most amazing bit of driving I've ever seen.

An hour later and we're safely anchored in Cornwallis, with the *Rescue 1* crew coming aboard our vessel. Most don't say anything. They come aboard, shake our hands, and sit down with nervous smiles. The commodore is last to come aboard. He sits down, shaking his head in disbelief. Over the next hour we relive the horrifying night, recounting things from their side and our side, piecing the full story together. I'm just happy to be alive, having come so close to losing *Earthrace* and her crew.

The *Rescue 1* team leaves, and we head to bed in the ransacked sleeping quarters. None of us sleeps, though. Our minds continue to race, reliving the horrifying night over and over again. I'm also feeling a strong sense of guilt. Firstly, I foolishly went out in treacherous conditions with inexperienced crew, putting us all at risk. I then made the decision to come in over the notorious Manukau bar, when really we'd have been better off remaining in the relative safety of deep water. I risked not only our lives, but also the lives of the gutsy Coastguard crew who selflessly came out to guide us over. Lastly, I'd headed into shallow water following what I'd thought was *Rescue 1*, and it turned out to be a light on shore. All up, a dreadful performance. When the storm forecast came in I'd been keen to test out *Earthrace*, thinking little about the dangers involved. I'd been taught a real lesson. The only good thing was that we made it through the ordeal with no loss of life.

I start to have second thoughts about *Earthrace*. It had all seemed so easy in the beginning. Build a boat, fuel it on biodiesel, and set a new world record for a powerboat to circumnavigate the globe. I didn't reckon on anything like the harrowing experience we'd just had, and we haven't even left New Zealand yet.

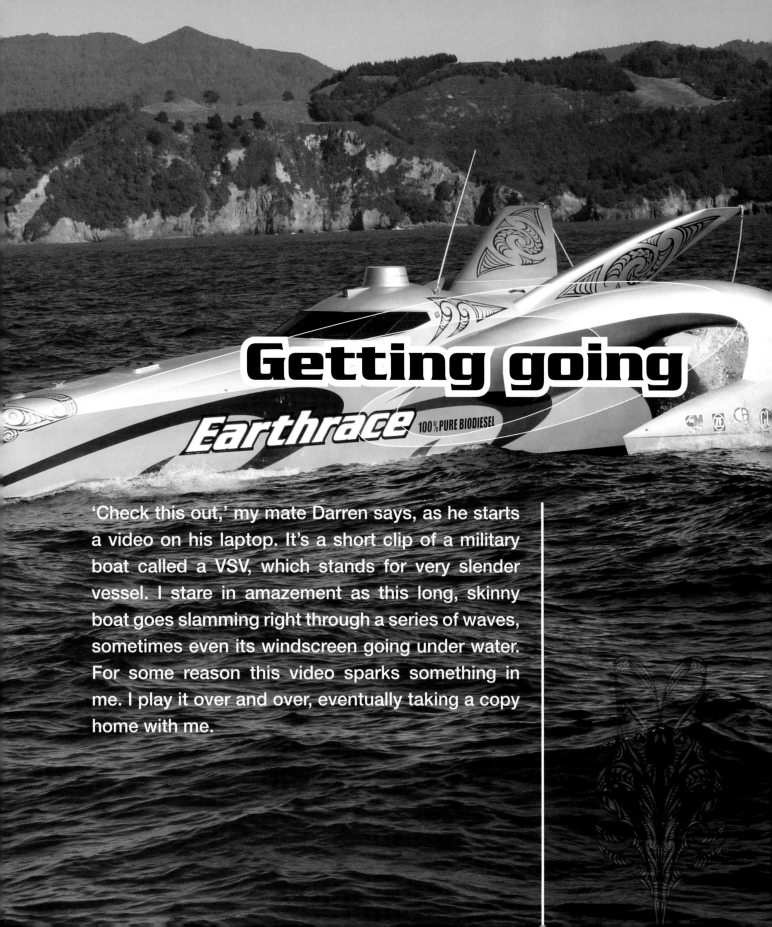

# Getting going

'Check this out,' my mate Darren says, as he starts a video on his laptop. It's a short clip of a military boat called a VSV, which stands for very slender vessel. I stare in amazement as this long, skinny boat goes slamming right through a series of waves, sometimes even its windscreen going under water. For some reason this video sparks something in me. I play it over and over, eventually taking a copy home with me.

For the next couple of months, I begin learning all I can about these unique boats, gradually becoming more and more engrossed in the technology. There are several keys to their performance. The bows are very narrow, in some cases almost chisel shaped, giving them very little buoyancy in the forward section. So when they hit a wave, the bow tends to cleave it apart and pass through, rather than rising up and over like a normal boat. In some boats there is also a ballast tank in the forward section that they fill with water. This added weight further reduces bow buoyancy, increasing the amount of piercing.

In flat water the wave-piercing boat offers nothing special, and in fact a conventional deep V design is perhaps slightly better. In rough seas, however, a wave-piercer will keep a flatter trajectory, reducing stresses on both the vessel and the crew. This in turn allows the vessel to be driven faster.

A large number of these boats are single-hull military vessels, and they're mostly used for getting SAS troops from A to B as quickly as possible. One version, around 56 feet long, is actually made to fit inside a C131 transport aeroplane, sometimes being dropped at sea attached to parachutes. Apparently, one boat in 10 that gets dropped doesn't make it back! There are also some partial wave-piercing boats in the form of fast ferries, although these have only the pontoons piercing water. Overall, however, there are virtually no pleasure boats, charter boats or race boats employing this technology.

What about building a wave-piercing boat for diving and fishing? I wonder one day over breakfast. It'd mean I could get out on rough days when you'd normally just stay at home. It'd also get to the spots quicker. More time fishing, less time travelling. So I'm busy hatching a plan for a relatively small wave-piercer, when I stumble onto the website of Union Internationale Motonautique (UIM), the certifying authority for powerboat records. As I scan the list, one record leaps out at me. It's one for a powerboat to circumnavigate the globe and, amazingly, it's almost 75 days, which is even longer than many yachts take. It looks like a record there for the taking.

As I'm pondering the record, it strikes me that a wave-piercer would be an ideal boat for going around the globe. In such a long voyage, statistically you're bound to get a few storms with rough seas, and in these conditions a wave-piercer would be favoured.

It seems odd, though, that I should suddenly start to think much about boats, as I've never really been into them. I've had a six-metre aluminium runabout for around 10 years, but it's just been a means to go diving or fishing, and a necessary evil in order to get to good spots. Not that I hated my time on the water, but that was always secondary to catching fish or grabbing some scallops and a few crays. Which is the same as many Kiwis, I suspect. So it was weird how I should suddenly find myself engrossed in wave-piercing boats, spending most of my spare time learning about them.

The other thing that happened around this time was I became a real convert to biodiesel fuel. To complete my Master of Business Administration in Sydney, I'd written a 20,000-word thesis titled 'Alternative Fuels for Road Transport'.

# I'm lying there awake one night, thinking about all this, when it just dawns on me

Through this research, I became a real convert to biodiesel as a renewable fuel that can easily be integrated into road transport, and especially in countries like New Zealand. It has many advantages, both economic and environmental, and this has seen many governments, especially in Europe, adopt strong policies to support it. At the time, there was little progress in New Zealand, aside from a single company, Biodiesel Oils New Zealand, who were researching making biodiesel from tallow.

I'm lying there awake one night, thinking about all this, when it just dawns on me. Build a wave-piercing boat to attempt the round the world speed record, but fuel it with biodiesel, and run the whole project as a promotion for renewable fuels. How cool would that be? — and it just rolls off the tongue so easily when I explain it to Sharyn the next morning over breakfast.

'Well, why would you want to do that?' she replies after my long spiel. She stops pouring milk on her muesli and looks at me like I've lost my mind.

It's a good question, though. Why would you want to do it? If I was to just set the record running normal diesel, who would care? It'd just be a selfish exercise to get my name in the record books, not to mention a waste of resources. But to do it on biodiesel, that would be a fantastic positive promotion for renewable fuels. Not to mention a lot of fun.

Later that day I pop into Darren's boat building yard in Albany. I explain my plans to him, and he gives me that same 'you're mad' look that Sharyn had a few hours earlier. I can see he's curious, though, and pretty soon we're tracking down the details of all the wave-piercing boat designers. It turns out to be just a handful: one in Australia, one in the UK, one in Germany and, thankfully, one in New Zealand. The New Zealand designer is a guy by the name of Craig Loomes, and his team have won several awards recently, including one at the Fort Lauderdale boat show.

'I'd like you to design me a boat to go around the world in record time,' I say on my first meeting with Craig.

He raises his eyebrows at me. 'I want to fuel it on biodiesel. And I want it

# 'I'd like you to design me a boat to go around the world in record time'

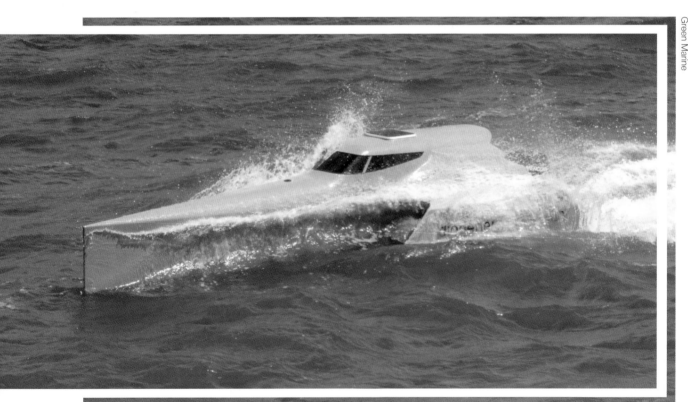

Green Marine

The 6.5 metre prototype during sea trials on the Hauraki Gulf.
It was an amazing little boat.

to be a wave-piercer.' He looks at me for a few moments then starts pulling up images on his PC of designs he's worked on recently.

'This one here,' he says enthusiastically, 'was developed for a fast ferry in Mauritius, but they still haven't gone ahead with it.' The design has three hulls, although the outside two look more like outriggers than full hulls. 'We believe it will be an outstanding boat for record attempts, but no one has ever built one of these before, so we're not 100 per cent sure what its performance will be like. What about something along those lines?' he asks, looking back over his shoulder at me.

The trouble is I know little about boats. All the words he and his team use mean little to me. Waterline length, sponsons, bulkheads, they roll off their tongues like I should know what they're saying, but I don't. I explain my situation to him, suggesting he'll need to guide me on the project for a while.

'I'd suggest we use this design then,' he says, pointing back at the image still on his PC screen, 'but we build a small prototype first to prove the concept.'

Darren and I then start wheeling and dealing to get a prototype built. The guy in Mauritius agrees to buy an outboard motor for it. Craig does the design for free. A few companies donate some odds and ends, and Darren agrees to build it at his yard, so long as he gets to keep the boat afterwards. This is fine by me, because all I need are the test results. The great thing with this arrangement is that the prototype gets built, but without costing me anything.

Six months later and Darren and I are down at Waiake Beach on Auckland's North Shore with the freshly painted 6.5 metre prototype. 'It looks like a James Bond boat, eh?' I say to Darren, as we're unhitching it from the trailer. The boat looks amazing, and in just a few minutes there's a crowd around us asking what we're up to. The Mercury outboard is fired up and I'm off, hooning around the sanctuary of the secluded bay. The ride feels rather spongy, with a tendency to porpoise. I'm actually thinking it's not that great, as I venture out into the open harbour.

There's a shallow reef protecting the bay from waves and as I go over it, I'm suddenly faced with a fat one-and-a-half-metre wave coming directly at me. Let's see if this wave-piercing really works, I think, as I push the throttle wide open. I'm about to hit the wave, and feel I'm going too fast, but it's too late to back off. The boat launches into the wall of water, and there's an audible crack as the windscreen is engulfed. The cabin goes dark as the wave rolls over the top, and then it's suddenly all light again as we blast out the other side.

In that instant, I know that I'll make the record attempt in a wave-piercer. Any normal six-metre boat thrown at a wave like that would be airborne for several seconds, before it and the crew crashed in a heap. I yell with joy, and spend the next while hunting waves and seeing how far under water I can get the little prototype. I pull back into Waiake Beach over an hour later where Darren is waiting. 'That boat is just unbelievable,' I gush to him and the few bystanders who are still hanging around. Darren clambers in and heads off, looking for waves. I stand there admiring the boat as it gradually disappears in the distance. It sure is an amazing-looking boat.

During the testing period that follows, numbers gradually come in confirming the design. 'What happens is the two sponsons are riding on the wake of the central hull, almost like surfing, and it makes the boat very efficient,' Loomes had explained to me. 'But it only happens over a certain speed range. For your record attempt, we'd need to optimise the surfing so it is maximised around your target speed.'

Buoyed by success of the prototype, work commences in earnest on a design for a full race boat. It starts off at around 30 metres in length, comes back to 20 metres, then up to 24 metres, as Craig and his team work through various design options. The goal is to have as small a boat as possible, which will minimise our total fuel consumed, but large enough that it still has a good chance of breaking the record. Some aspects of the prototype are not ideal, and the designers work to improve these. Some characteristics, like sponson surfing, are fantastic, and so these features are optimised or enhanced. This process is basically just Craig and his team working through it, and I have minimal involvement, given my limited knowledge of boats in general.

One aspect they do consult me on is the horns. I wander into their design office in Westhaven one morning, and Craig asks what I think of his latest design. I look down at his PC screen and he's drawn in what could only be described as a snorkel — and it looks crap, which is pretty much what I tell him. 'The trouble we have,' explains Craig, 'is we need an easy way to ventilate the engine bay. We must get hot air out and cool air in, and it's not so easy to do on a boat that submarines.' Even so, I still can't see me driving a boat with ugly snorkels on top. 'Leave it to me, I'll work on it,' he says confidently at the end of our meeting. There follows a series of emails as he works through different options. The ventilation goes from a snorkel to a rooster tail, to vertical horns, and then these gradually work back to a pair of curved horns.

It is an interesting lesson in how the design process works. Craig comes up with a shape, but then Andre, Rupert or other members of his team work on fitting this around existing structures, determine how the components can be built, and evaluate whether it all stacks up. It is a repetitive process, backwards and forwards, with gradual refinements as the design is fine-tuned. Even so, the horns polarise people. In the end I like them, but I figure there are other people better at deciding such things. 'You're the expert, you do the design and I'll just go with it,' is my parting comment to Craig.

A month or so later, and the design has evolved into a truly amazing shape. If I thought the prototype looked good, the full race boat looks unbelievable. With my limited input, Craig and his team have had free rein

Craig Loomes Design Group

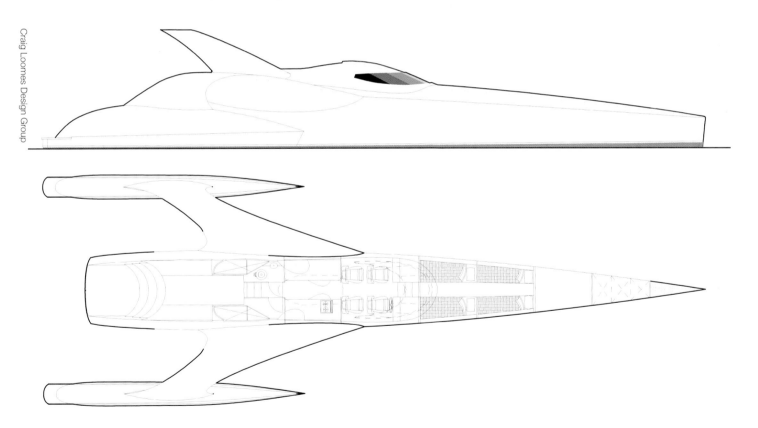

CAD drawing of *Earthrace*.

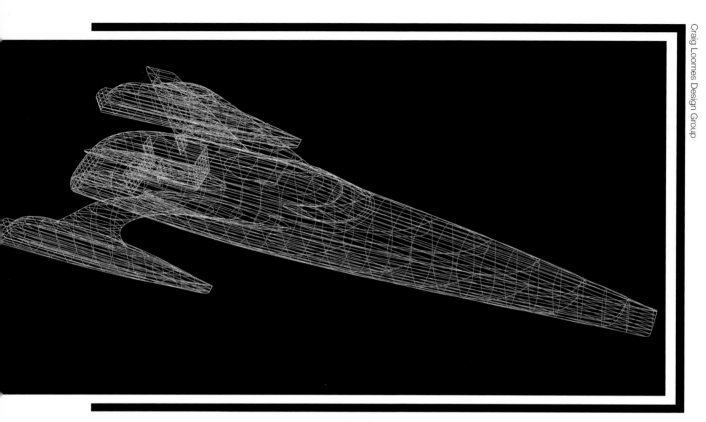

CAD drawing of *Earthrace*.

to do whatever they liked, and the end result is a reflection of giving them this freedom. Most people getting boats designed try to squeeze as much living space as they can into the size of vessel they can afford. In so doing, however, they also force the designer into conventional square boxes, which may be the most efficient in space, but not necessarily the best in other respects. That's why most boats look the same: a single hull, a series of square boxes on top and painted white.

There's another reason boats have a tendency to look alike: the marine industry is very unforgiving. Faulty designs show up in boats that spectacularly fall apart, sometimes even with loss of life. As a result, naval architects have become a conservative breed, and especially in countries such as the United States with a very litigious population. Their designs follow tried and proven formulae with low risk. What has worked in the past will continue to work in the future.

In New Zealand, however, our legislation is such that high proof of negligence is required in order to sue someone. This has given our designers slightly more freedom in developing new designs and innovations. Also, our marine industry has become extremely innovative in order to survive. Our home market is relatively small, especially when it comes to larger boats, and so local designers are continually trying new and unproven concepts, some of which become highly successful, in order to get noticed in competitive overseas markets.

I'm admiring the latest set of CAD files on our kitchen table when Sharyn wanders in, and starts looking through the pages.

'How much is this all going to cost?' she finally asks, as she turns the last page over.

'About three million dollars.'

'And where exactly will you get three million dollars from?'

'Well, I'm not sure yet, but I reckon I'll ask for four.'

Which is exactly what I've started doing. Over the last couple of weeks I've been contacting all the large businesses I can track down, to see if they're interested in sponsoring us. The hope is to have one of them give us enough money to run the whole project, which on initial budgets appears to be around three million bucks.

The task, though, is much harder than I'd first thought. I really need to meet with either the heads of these big businesses or, as a second choice, their marketing or communications managers. The challenge is that these people often have layers of staff protecting them from people like me. 'Send us a proposal and I'll forward it to Mr Jones,' is a typical response, but I never hear back, despite spending days chasing them on the phone. In some instances I do get to talk to the right person, but the rejections are pretty fast in coming.

'What about looking overseas?' Steve Adams says to me after another disappointing week of cold calling and pointless phone calls. Steve has agreed to work free for me to get the project going, and with his background in PR and sponsorship, he's shedding some light on how we should be packaging the project. 'I reckon you should be looking in the US or Europe where there's a lot more sponsorship money floating around — and you need to come up with a decent name.' He's right on both counts, I figure. The sort of money we need really requires a global brand, and there are only a handful of those in New Zealand, who by now are likely sick of my calls. As for the name, something a little more inspiring would be nice.

'What about *Earthrace*?' Steve asks in an email the next day. 'You're racing around the earth. There is also a race towards sustainability to save the planet, of which biodiesel is a key component.' I Google 'Earthrace' and get 18 hits. Some guy by the name of Tom Keene has written a book called *Earthrace*, but aside from that the name is unused. So *Earthrace* it is.

We spend a month fine-tuning our proposals. A company isn't going to give us money because we're nice or because we have a good-looking boat.

'They will only give us money if it helps them sell more products or services,' Steve explains to me. So we work on specifics about what we can offer. TV news items, TV series, DVDs, website traffic, books, magazines, radio interviews, posters, T-shirts, direct sales, hospitality, promotional events, signage, all may have interest to potential sponsors. The challenge we have is that we don't really know how much the full project will cost, but we need to at least come up with some numbers. So we make some rough estimates and go with it. The budget is set at US$4m, of which a million is set aside for promotions.

## They will only give us money if it helps them sell more products or services

We then start organising a sales trip to the US and Europe. Coca-Cola, Pepsi, Vodafone, Red Bull, Ford, General Motors, Volkswagen, Peugeot, Sprint. We start hassling all of them. 'Don't sell the project, sell the meeting,' Steve advises me. Trying to get meetings with these companies isn't easy, but some do agree. Gradually, the schedule unfolds, with two weeks planned in the US and 10 days in Europe. We don't have all the meetings organised, but some we see as key we'll keep working on during the trip. 'Don't come back without a cheque,' Sharyn says, dropping me off at Auckland International Airport.

My flights are from Auckland to Los Angeles then connecting to New York, where the first few meetings are arranged. On the flight to New York, I'm sitting next to a guy who takes up his own seat and half of mine. 'These seats are just way too small,' he says to me with a thick Southern drawl, as he's adjusting his seat belt. He's so big the air hostess has given him an extension for the seat belt. I'm thinking of telling him he should get a business class seat. He sneezes, his big belly shuddering against my side.

I normally make a point of talking to the people next to me on flights. Over the years I've met some really interesting people, so I make a start with this guy. 'What are you up to in New York?' I ask, as the air hostesses move past, closing the overhead compartments.

'Oh I'm working on a communications strategy for one of our clients.' I'm thinking maybe his client could use a boat to help with this. 'Who's the client?'

He looks at me for a few seconds, as if deciding whether to answer. He says, eventually, in slightly hushed tones, 'We're looking to make nuclear energy more accepted in America.' Now, as an engineer, and without giving it much thought, I've always been kind of keen on nuclear energy. So I get him talking about it. 'The good thing with nuclear energy,' he points out, 'is there are no emissions and no greenhouse gases. You're not dependent on the weather, unlike wind and hydro generation . . . and the only resource you consume is a tiny amount of uranium.'

'Well, if it is so good, how come they need to employ you to make it acceptable?' I figure I already know the answer.

Bob, it seems, has given this talk many times. 'Do you realise,' he continues, getting slightly animated now, 'if the average US citizen had all the energy they consume through their lifetime, so this includes their transport, electricity, heating, everything, if it is all derived from nuclear energy, at the end of their life they'd only account for nuclear waste the size of a tennis ball?' Which is actually quite amazing, I have to admit. The plane starts to accelerate down the runway, and Bob suddenly grabs the two armrests and braces himself. 'I hate flying,' he says, gritting his teeth. I look up at his face and he's sweating profusely.

A while later and he's settled down a bit, the plane now just in a gentle climb. 'Well, what do you do with the waste?' I ask.

'Most of it gets solidified, sealed up in canisters and stored. Today there are over a hundred sites around the US safely storing waste fuel, but once the Yucca Mountain complex is complete, it'll all be stored in Nevada.'

'And how long do you need to store it for?'

Bob looks at me again for a few moments before answering. 'Oh, only a few thousand years.' There's a long silence between us. Bob finally fills the gap. 'Which isn't that long when you consider the advantages.'

I sit there mulling this over for a while. The thought of people having to store nuclear waste for the next two thousand years because of energy we consume today is appalling. Imagine how we'd feel if we were forced to store waste products from people who'd lived two thousand years ago. There's also the issue of where you store it. Maybe the people in Nevada are OK with storing all the US nuclear waste on their doorstep, but I sure wouldn't be. Nuclear energy doesn't seem so appealing to me any more. Powering ourselves into the future is easy, but to do it in a sustainable way, and such that it doesn't pass our problems down through future generations sure isn't. Eventually, I drift off to sleep, squished between the armrest and Bob.

New York is one of those cities that polarises people. 'It's like a giant melting pot, where the scum eventually rises to the top,' someone had said to me once, which seems unfair really. There are some scum elements I guess, but there's also an energy and excitement about this city that is just intoxicating. It's a congested, bustling mass of people and buildings, where fortunes are won and lost in a short time. Sometimes it looks just like in the movies. As far as *Earthrace* goes, it's our best hope for finding a title sponsor.

I head into Manhattan by train, going over my presentation. The first meeting is only an hour away, and I look like crap after the flights, so I scurry into a KFC toilet to get sorted. I'm busy putting shaving gel on my face when a skinny black guy comes in and tries selling me drugs. 'Anyfink ya want I kin git,' he says to me in a gangsta-like voice. His eyes are yellow, and his head moves in a series of twitches. 'Yo, what yafta?'

'Um, no thanks mate. I just need to get shaved and tidied up,' I reply nervously. He looks at me curiously.

'Wher yiz from?'

'From New Zealand,' I say, running the razor down my right cheek.

'Ho, Noooo Zeeeland.' I'm watching him in the mirror and I can see him eyeing up my pack lying on the floor. His head twitches back to look at me then he disappears out the door.

My Waikato rugby jersey is swapped for a suit, which has survived its journey in my pack surprisingly well. As I wander out the KFC door, I see the drug dealer waiting in the carpark. 'Anyfink yiz afta,' he yells over at me. I smile and give him a wave, hurrying off for my appointment just a block away.

It's a towering glass building, with a reception area like a hotel lobby. I leave my pack with the security guards and catch an elevator up to floor 56.

'Tell me about recent record attempts,' Tara says to me towards the end of the meeting. I talk a little about *Cable & Wireless*, the existing record holder, and mention there have been some attempts since, but none of them has taken the record.

'What happened to them?' she asks. It's as if she knows the answer. Since 1998 there have been four other record attempts, but none has finished. Two of the boats have actually sunk. It's an awkward area, and I know it will deter many companies from sponsoring us, if they think there is a 50 per cent chance of us sinking, and only a 50 per cent chance of us actually finishing. The meeting ends shortly afterwards, and I wander out thinking I need to make a better job of talking about past record attempts.

Over the following two weeks, it's meeting upon meeting, with some organisations committing to take it further, but none that really grab the project and run with it.

I'm starting to feel I lack the sales skills to pull this off. It's brought home to me, believe it or not, by a trip to McDonald's. On the breakfast menu is this thing called an Egg McMuffin, something I've never had before, so I ask the lad at the counter what it's like.

'Oh, it's just fantastic! It's got these fresh eggs, cooked just right, and these beautiful buns toasted just the way you like them.' He waxes lyrical about how great they are, then asks if I'd like one or two. So I get two of them, of course. They turn out to be awful, and I end up eating just one.

It highlights for me something about Americans. They are such wonderful salespeople, and it's drilled into them from an early age. Us Kiwis, by contrast, well, we tend to undersell ourselves. The guy in McDonald's could make his Egg McMuffin sound more exciting than my taking a boat around the globe. Here I am in the most competitive country on earth, trying to sell a project for four million bucks, and I'm up against an army of people all selling projects, and probably all doing a much better job of it.

I'm pondering this as I fly out from JFK Airport on my way to Europe. I need to get better at selling the Earthrace concept, not by misleading people, but by making them realise what an awesome project it will be, and how it will help their brand. I also need to do better in getting appointments with senior executives. In the US, many appointments were with people well down the food chain, most of whom have little or no influence in their companies. The European trip coming up is disjointed. Over the 10 days I'm visiting five countries and attending 16 meetings. I land in Munich and hire a rental car. 'You know ve drive on za uzza side of za road here,' the lady at the Hertz counter says to me. She's got that stern, matronly look about her, like one of my old school teachers.

'Yeah yeah, just give me the keys,' I reply cheekily, extending out my hand. She hands over the keys while looking down her long, Aryan nose at me. 'Ze car is parked zere,' she says, pointing at a row of white cars outside the window. Grabbing my pack I wander outside, and start looking along the row of cars. I find mine on the end, unlock it with the remote, and jump in. To my amusement, I'm sitting in the passenger seat. In Germany, like the lady had said, they drive on the right-hand side of the road. I look up and there is the Hertz matron standing in the window with one hand on her hip and the other wagging a finger accusingly at me, like I've been caught drinking behind the bike-shed. I jump out laughing, and scamper around to the driver's side.

One company I'm especially keen on meeting here is Volkswagen, who in the past have been very supportive of biodiesel initiatives. Their marketing manager has resisted agreeing to a meeting, so I've decided to just turn up on his doorstep in Wolfsburg. Despite reaching speeds of 200 kilometres an hour along the autobahn, it's still after 2am before I arrive there. A quick scout around town reveals only a couple of open hotels, with rates over 250 euros for a single night — and I'll only need the room for a few hours. Eventually, I decide to sleep in the car and save my money. It's a cold winter night, though, and I wake up every half hour or so to turn the engine on and warm myself up.

At sparrow's fart next morning I'm at the guardhouse of the Wolfsburg assembly plant. The marketing manager is not at work yet. Then word comes down that he has arrived, but has a busy schedule, and may not be able to meet with me. I have no other appointments today anyway, so I just hang around talking to the guard, on the off chance that I can get in for a meeting. At six in the evening I give up. I hop in my rental and start the long drive to Fulda, where I have an appointment the following morning. It's been a depressing day.

Over the next two weeks, Europe follows a similar pattern to the US: lots of meetings with people agreeing what a cool project it is, but none really jumping at the chance to get involved. A few agree to look further at it, though, and there's a steady trickle of emails going backwards and forwards. A couple of US companies also remain interested but, again, nothing solid. I board my flight from Heathrow back to Auckland, not really knowing what to do from here, other than simply following up with the few positive leads that are left.

A month later and one company has become increasingly interested in the project. As we exchange emails, I'm starting to think they really will come in and be our title sponsor. One aspect they are focusing on is the promotional tour through North America before the record attempt. By stopping in different cities for a few days, they see it as a chance to get local TV and newspaper coverage, while also providing some great hospitality opportunities for local distributors. They'll have their products on display, effectively making it a travelling road show around coastal cities in the US and Canada.

# 'There's only one problem left and that's this biodiesel fuel. It just doesn't fit our brand'

'These guys will sign up,' I say to Sharyn confidently one morning as I'm working on an email back to them.

'Well, someone had better sign up soon,' she replies. 'There's only fifteen hundred bucks left in our account and our mortgage comes out next week.' The Earthrace project has recently started to look like a black hole. I worked out the other day we'd spent almost $70,000 already, and all we have to show for it are a bunch of proposals and a few emails. I hit the send button and my email beams off into cyberspace.

A few days later and I'm finalising details with their marketing manager, confident of wrapping up the deal. 'Look Pete, the promotional tour is great. The money you're needing is fine.' I'm starting to think this is the moment when they write me a big fat cheque.

'There's only one problem left and that's this biodiesel fuel. It just doesn't fit our brand.'

There's a long pause while I digest what he's saying. Biodiesel fuel is the reason I'm doing this. Finally, he says, 'If you could run the project on normal diesel we'd be a lot more comfortable.' He's basically offering me four million bucks, but only if we get rid of the biodiesel.

It's not like I'd ever consider running the project on normal diesel.

Like I've said it'd just turn into a selfish exercise to get my name in the record books. I despondently send an email off to Steve, letting him know what's happened, when Sharyn walks in. She can see straight away that I'm disappointed about something. I explain to her the offer we have. 'You're not accepting, are you?' she says, suddenly worried I'm about to sell my soul. We talk late into the night about what we should do. In the end we agree to give it another month, and if we haven't signed a sponsor by then, we'll flag the project away.

A week's gone by with nothing bright on the horizon, when there's an unexpected call from a guy at Cummins Mercruiser in Charleston, South Carolina. He's heard about Earthrace through the grapevine, and wants to get involved as a sponsor. So I pack my bags and head off to America again, this time with one big, fat appointment in my diary.

'Tell me about Earthrace,' Gary Dickman says shortly after I walk into his office. He's got that nasally twang of an Australian I'm thinking, as I launch into my usual spiel. Gary eventually cuts me off.

'What size engines do you need?'

'Umm, about 500 horsepower.'

# 'I can't give you four million bucks, but I can sponsor you two engines for the race'

Gary starts going into details of their new QSC engine, which puts out about 540 horsepower. Lightweight, super-efficient, and it meets the tier-2 emission standards. Sounds perfect, I'm thinking.

'I can't give you four million bucks,' Gary finally says, 'but I can sponsor you two engines for the race. We'll service them and provide you all the spare parts and consumables you need, and at the end of the programme we'll rebuild them for you.'

I sit there considering his offer. Two free engines. I'd be a mug not to accept them. It cuts down how much sponsorship we'll need. So we shake hands on it. *Earthrace* now has two engines on the way. I'm just about to leave when Gary has a thought.

'You'll need some gearboxes, won't you?' Actually I have no idea if we need them or not. The designers mentioned two engines, but no one said anything about gearboxes.

'Yes,' I respond, not wanting to sound ignorant.

'Look, we know the guys at ZF Marine really well. Leave it to me and we'll sort out a couple of sponsored gearboxes for you as well.'

How cool is that? I leave Charleston having sorted two engines and two gearboxes. It has started me thinking I don't need four million bucks from one company to make this happen. Maybe we can piece it together with a range of smaller sponsorships. The engine and gearbox sponsorships fell into place so easily, maybe others will be like that as well.

So I decide to just go scrounging for hardware and services we'll need for the boat. With Cummins and ZF Marine on board it has given us some credibility, so companies seem much more willing to support us. I had no success at getting cash, but getting freebies for the boat is easy. Navman jump on board with electronics, 3M the signwriting materials, Pilkington Glass the windscreens, Ameron the paint.

'Check this out,' I say to Sharyn, as I'm busy updating the sponsors list. 'We now have over 1.5 million dollars' worth of goods and services sponsored.' It's an impressive list, with over a hundred companies contributing.

'How much more do you need?' she replies, looking around our lounge, now resembling a marine chandlery store.

'Well, I reckon that is about all of it, with the exception of carbon and labour. But I'm thinking we'll just have to pay for them anyway.'

Carbon has remained difficult. In fact we're struggling to even find the carbon for construction, let alone getting it sponsored. There's a global shortage, caused firstly by military demand for things like APC vehicles, now all getting blown to bits in Iraq, and secondly by the aerospace industry, which is increasingly building carbon frames rather than aluminium.

As for the labour, I've visited all the major yards and a few small ones, promoting the project, and looking for a really sharp deal. Calibre Boats, a new yard with some outstanding boat builders, have offered to build the boat at cost — which is about as good a deal as I think we'll get. It could have us starting construction in a few months, funds permitting.

'And where are the funds going to come from?' Sharyn asks.

'Well, to get started, we could sell off our shares and unit trusts. We could sell our stake in CamSensor, and we could sell the forestry block. We could also throw a mortgage on the house.'

Sharyn looks over at me, with a frown on her face. 'There's no way we're parting with the forestry block. It's our retirement plan, remember?' She sits down next to me. 'Are you sure you really want to go ahead with this?'

We're at the crossroads right now. Once we start, we're fully committed to the project, and will need to come up with a substantial chunk of money to make it happen. Even with the funds I'm talking of putting in, Earthrace will require much, much more. I now really believe in the project, however, and I believe we can make a substantial contribution towards promoting renewable fuels. For me, I'm not really fussed about the money. It is only money, after all. How can I expect others to put in funds if I'm not prepared to do so myself?

The irony here is most of the money we're looking to put in has come from the oil industry. On completing my engineering degree at Auckland University, I was employed by an amazing company called Schlumberger as a wireline engineer. The company is involved in the high-tech area of oil exploration, and the job saw me running operations on oil rigs in the North Sea and North Africa, logging some major production fields, as well as being involved in discovering some new ones. The experience gave me a solid understanding of fossil fuels, where we find them, and what it takes to get them out of the ground. I also made a truckload of money in a short time, a large chunk of it about to go into *Earthrace*.

The hardest asset to cash in will be CamSensor, a company I co-founded with a couple of other engineers some six years ago. We make cameras for automated quality control on production lines, and more recently in guiding robots, but there are so few potential purchasers of shares in such a small and specialised company. It's also a shame to sell something you've spent so much of your time building up. I've started asking around, though, and we'll see what offers turn up. As *Earthrace* has progressed I've found myself working less and less at CamSensor anyway, and it'll probably be a relief to sell my shares and just go full-time on the boat, albeit without pay. We'll see what offers turn up anyway.

With the detailed design of *Earthrace* completed, Craig Ross, the owner of Calibre Boats, gets to work on budgets. Construction labour comes in at $300k under what we'd originally expected. The carbon estimate is also well down. This is good news when you've just taken out a mortgage on your house to help with funding. The proposed start date for construction is February 2005, which should see us launched around August.

'If you're starting construction, you really need a cameraman to film it,' Steve says to me. 'If you can film the whole story, you'll be able to sell a series to Discovery channel, which will help us raise sponsorship.' I think about this for a while. There's no way I can afford to pay someone to film construction yet. If Steve's prepared to work for no pay, though, maybe other people will as well. Actually, there's probably a whole range of jobs we could flick out to people if they're prepared to work for free.

There starts from here a programme we later called Earthrace Volunteers. The first to sign up is a talented young filmmaker by the name of Ryan Heron. We meet for a couple of hours and he agrees to do whatever filming we need. Next we place an online advert requesting a volunteer photographer. Within a couple of days we have over 50 applications. From this we pick the top five to interview and we choose Tim Costar to join our team.

The surprising thing is how easy it was to get these people on board. All I offered was the chance to contribute, and there was suddenly a queue of people all wanting to get involved. It highlights for me attitudes of many young people. I don't know why or how, but we have somehow raised a generation of kids who really do give a toss about the environment. While my generation focuses on getting a bigger house, a four-wheel drive, plasma TVs and a stainless refrigerator, these young adults are busy wondering what they can do to help the environment — and they're prepared to work without pay, given the right cause. I guess they're also interested in where the next party will be, but you can hardly blame them for that.

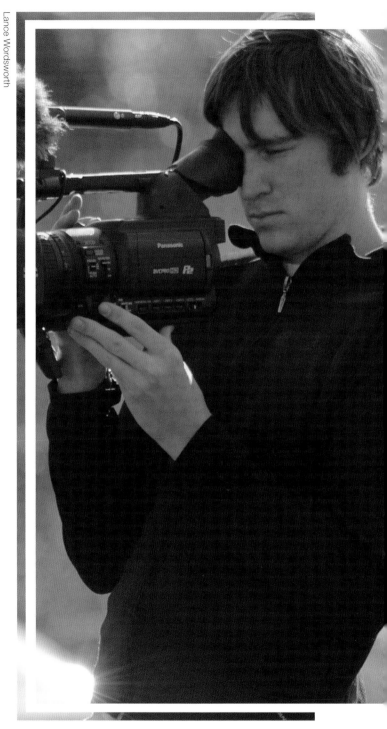

Lance Wordsworth

Ryan filming.

# Construction gets under way

Before we know it February has arrived and construction begins, although I still know virtually nothing about the building process. I've spent the last six months tying up sponsorships for goods and services to be used in construction, with little understanding on how each would be used.

'What do ya reckon?' says Calibre's head boat builder Tony Clayton as I wander into the yard. I look around and the shed is just vacant space, which in a few months will gradually fill with *Earthrace*. Right now, the only progress is a few bits of board bolted to the floor, and a few marks on top.

'Man, it's just wicked to be under way,' I say to Tony.

Construction of most sections is relatively simple. It starts with sheets of medium density fibreboard (MDF) that have been laser cut in profile, and are lined up in a row. Into this, the boat builders lay sections of foam and bend them into the shape defined by the sheets of MDF. The foam is stuck in place with resins. Once it has set in the basic shape, carbon will be laminated on the inside of the foam. When this has dried, the foam-carbon piece is relatively rigid, and can be removed from the mould. Carbon and other materials will then be laminated on the outside. This is called sandwich composites. You have foam, 40 millimetres thick in this case, sandwiched between layers of carbon and other fibres. It results in a super -light structure that, if well made, is also extremely strong.

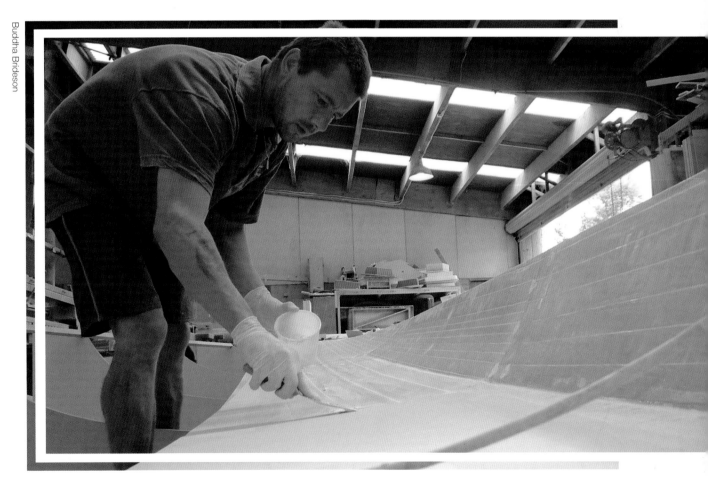

Buddha Brideson

Tony Clayton working on the inside of the port sponson during early construction.

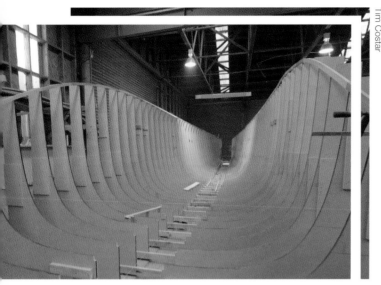

*Tim Costar*

Looking down what we called the whale carcass. The MDF sheets are laser cut then laid up in profile as you see here, along the length of the boat. The next step is to fit foam into this.

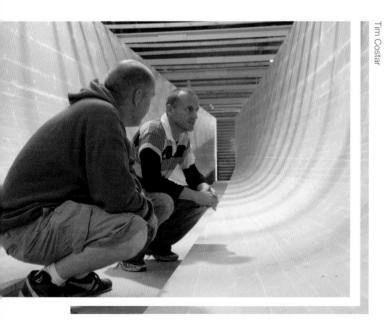

*Tim Costar*

Inside the main hull looking towards the bow. At this stage the hull is foam only, and the carbon is about to be laminated onto the inside.

'Here's your first load of black gold,' says Craig, lifting up a roll of carbon. 'There's about ten thousand bucks' worth in there,' he says, pointing at a small pallet of rolls on the floor. It comes as a cloth material, and is then made rigid with resins that will set, binding the fibres together. It has 10 times the strength to weight ratio of steel, and if you want to build something that is strong and light, carbon is the best option. Amazing stuff, really.

This structure has one drawback, though — it is relatively brittle. Some people liken a full carbon boat to one made entirely of glass (not the fibreglass type either). It is fantastic, as long as there are no flaws in it. But as soon as you get a chip or a crack, the vessel is likely to shatter, which in fact happened to a number of early carbon boats. The solution is to add the synthetic fibre Kevlar on the outside of the carbon. Kevlar is heavier than carbon, but has fantastic impact resistance properties. If the vessel does hit a log, for example, Kevlar localises the damage to a small area, rather than allowing the cracks to propagate.

The composite mix on the outside is finished with a thin E-glass layer for cross-axial strength, whatever that means, and finally fairing compound, which is like car bog. Fairing compound adds weight with little gain, other than ensuring a smooth boat, so considerable effort is made to have the boat fair to begin with, reducing the volume of fairing compound required. The end result of all this is a boat that is extremely light, that can handle some impacts without sinking, and can tolerate the enormous forces involved in submarining through waves. Or so the theory goes anyway.

The number of boat builders working on *Earthrace* gradually increases, and with it progress. The starboard sponson is nearly completed, and a second team then starts on the port sponson. I turn up at the yard on the day they're getting things in position for the central hull. Pallets of MDF sheets cut by North Shore Laser Cutters are lying next to the rolling door. The guys start at one end of the shed, standing up two matching half frames, getting them vertical then bracing them in position. By the end of the day, there are 55 frames all in a line. It is starting to look like a boat.

'You know, it's heaps bigger than I'd imagined,' Ryan says, as we're wandering down between the sheets. It almost feels like we're inside the boat and it is certainly imposing. Actually, it looks kind of like a whale carcass. We stop in the middle and attempt some filming, but it's just too dark to get a decent image. We flag it away and head outside to have a beer with the lads. 'It's a big bugger, isn't it?' Tony says to me, between mouthfuls of Speight's.

He's standing in front of the barbecue poking sausages and wild venison steaks with his spare hand. There are a few hunters in the group and there's normally something feral or aquatic cooking on the barbecue. Last Friday it was scallops and snapper. I grab a small chunk of venison and clench it between my teeth, allowing it to cool a bit before chewing. It's got that wild whiff that comes from animals eating leaves and other plant life from the wild. It's a good life we have in New Zealand, I reckon.

Craig brings out a couple of slabs of beer and throws them on the ground. 'Free beer, anyone?' A few murmurs and grunts of support emanate from the group. These guys sure like their beer. They have a page on the fridge with their name, a column for each day, and they place a tick each time they take a beer. By the end of the week there's an impressive row of marks next to most of their names. There's now a row for *Earthrace*, and a couple of ticks for the beers Ryan and I are drinking.

I look around the group, most of them sitting back in $5 Warehouse chairs. There's a certain contentedness about them — beer in hand and eagerly waiting on their steaks after a hard week of work. They're a rough and ready bunch as well. No *Cleo* centrefolds here, that's for sure, but good honest Kiwi blokes. Guys like this make up the backbone of boat building in New Zealand — practical, hard-working, good attention to detail, and fit and agile enough to get into confined spaces. Not an easy job, but also not that stressful. At the end of the day they go home, leaving their work

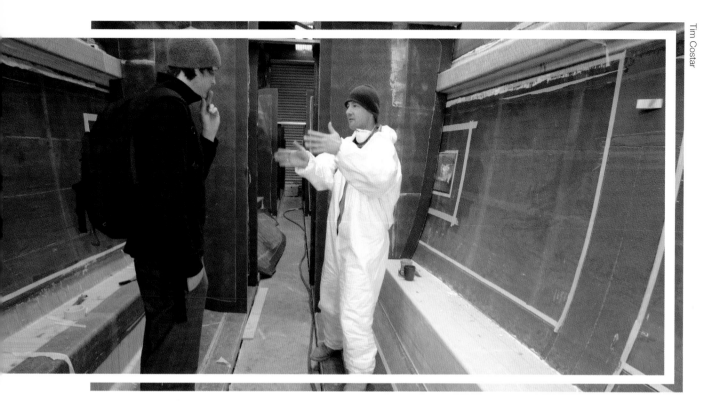

Tim Costar

Tony Clayton explains the process to Ryan Heron. The two half shells were made with a gap between them. We then winched the two halves together.

behind. I think about my current predicament with funds disappearing at an alarming rate, and nothing significant coming in.

Sponsorship has remained a difficult challenge. I continue to get dialogue with companies, and am getting a few of them interested, but most remain sceptical about our ability to get media attention. 'What makes you think TV networks will come and cover your boat?' the vice president of marketing for a bank had said to me the previous week. I explained to him that we had already been on TV a few times, that by doing the tour through North America we'd get TV there before the race, and then during the race they'd probably cover us because there is a local connection. We were also putting together a TV series, and we'd have a cameraman permanently aboard the boat to get race footage. It seems these people hear such stories all the time, though, and in the end he just wishes us good luck.

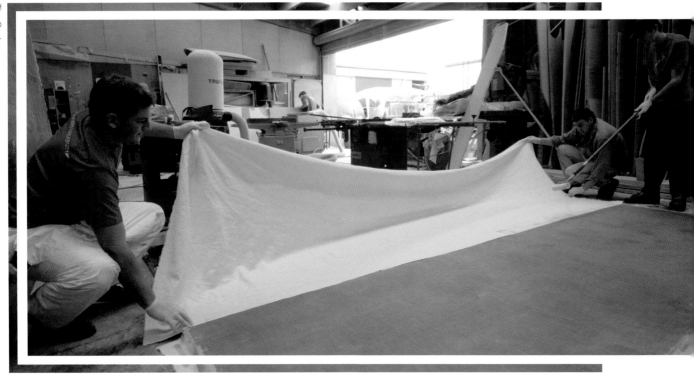

Gareth Beckermann from Waikato University, with Geoff and Tim Costar laying up hemp onto the floor sole. *Earthrace* is the first boat in the world to use hemp composite in construction.

'Banks are just too conservative anyway,' Steve says to me after listening to the call. 'We really need brands that are a bit edgy, rather than conservative — like an energy drink, or a beer company. Hey what about 42 Below?'

They would probably be a good fit, although they tend to just do media stunts, which are cheap compared with what we're looking to do. You never know, though. I look them up on the Internet and make a note to call them in the morning.

The following day 42 Below are a disappointment, but I do manage to sell my shares in CamSensor — for nothing like what the company is really worth, but at least I manage to cash them in. Our house has also had a new valuation, which is enabling us to increase our mortgage again. I'm barely off the phone talking with my bank manager, when an email arrives from Calibre Boats. 'Unless all payments are brought up to date by this Friday, we will cease work on *Earthrace*,' it says in capital letters. I'm not even a week late, and given his terms are only seven days, I'm feeling he's being a bit harsh. Especially when I've also paid him a $20k deposit.

The phone then rings from a mate. 'Pete, I just heard the news that work has stopped on *Earthrace* because you've not paid the workers.' Word was spreading that *Earthrace* was doomed.

When you cannot pay wages, everyone hears about it in such a small industry. Minutes later and the local newspaper calls wanting details.

It brings to focus our need to get some money fast. The money raised from CamSensor and the mortgage will keep us going for another month or so, but that is it. I start looking back over what we have achieved in terms of sponsors. It seems Steve and I are just no good at getting big companies to sponsor us with cash. Either that or they perceive too much risk in committing to such a new and unproven team. With the exception, of course, being the company who previously offered $4m, if we dropped the biodiesel fuel.

It's Friday night and I've cooked Sharyn dinner. Spaghetti bolognaise and a big fat rum and coke. Sharyn swallows all but the last mouthful from our shared glass, meaning I'll finish it and have to get up for the refill. We're lounging on the girls' beanbags and slinging ideas around. 'What about just borrowing the money,' Sharyn finally says. 'At least you'd be able to get the boat launched, and then you'll probably find it easier to attract sponsors.'

'Yeah, but who's going to loan me money for a boat?'

'Just start going through the rich list.'

It's an interesting idea. The 'rich list', in book form, clearly details the wealthiest people in the country, their background and a few of their business interests.

'Yeah, maybe. I'll give it a go next week and see how we get on.'

Some of the people are easy to track down, and within a few days I'm talking with the likes of David Richwhite, Peter Maire, Barry Coleman, Colin Giltrap and Roger Douglas. Mike Moore even gets involved. I also spend a few evenings door knocking along Paritai Drive in Remuera, arguably the wealthiest street in New Zealand. Cold calling such lavish houses can be an intimidating experience. In the end only two people give me more than about 30 seconds. One was a Malaysian Chinese lady who gave me an hour of her time and a couple of beers, but then felt it wasn't something she and her husband could support. There was also a man from Dubai who offered to charter the boat once launched.

In terms of funds, though, my efforts on the rich list and in Paritai Drive netted a big fat zero.

I only want a loan from them, but that seems as difficult as getting sponsorship.

Who can blame them? I'm just a cheeky little upstart wanting money for a boat after all.

Guys like Stephen Tindall and Sam Morgan must get thousands of people chasing them for money, and there are so many worthy causes out there all needing funds. It's worth the effort to give it a go, but I get the feeling I don't really connect well with this demographic.

# Who can blame them? I'm just a cheeky little upstart wanting money for a boat after all

There's also the thought in the back of my mind that some wealthy people are not that predisposed to environmental messages, because things like conserving resources go against their general ethos which is to consume or own as much as they can. If you look at it from a resource perspective, it is hard to justify having your own Lear jet, helicopter, or four-car garage. I visited a place in Portland, and the owner proudly proclaimed, 'My house has nine 50-inch plasma screens.' It was like I was supposed to be impressed. Well, let's say in the future legislation was passed limiting houses to say 200 square metres. How would such wealthy people respond to that I wonder? Or how about each family could own just one car? Or even your overseas holidays were limited to just one per year? All these would severely curtail lifestyles of the wealthy, and they'd surely be vociferous in resisting such measures.

The challenge, however, is we all need to find ways to reduce our consumption, but it's just harder for the wealthy because they have the most to give up. There are also, of course, a billion Chinese and a billion Indians all aspiring to the same levels of affluence as us. They all want to drive big cars, fly on international holidays and build big houses. Economically they can't do this right now, but what about in 100 years when their economies dwarf all, including the US?

I head back out to the boatyard, funding continuing to weigh heavily on me. It's an exciting day at the yard, though. The main hull is being flipped over, and there's a crew from TVNZ out filming it, as well as photographers from a couple of newspapers. The hull is loaded into cradles and pulled outside, where two cranes are waiting with slings. The hull is lifted, flipped over, then lowered back into the cradles.

'How's the money going Pete?' Craig enquires once the hull is back inside the shed.

'Not that good mate. I've got enough for one more week of construction, but that's it.' I look at Craig and I can see him weighing up his options. He must be wondering if we're going to go bust over this. We agree in the end to completing one more week of construction, after which they'll stop work on *Earthrace*.

Later that afternoon we get all the boat builders together and I give them the news. I can see there's disappointment on their faces. They were all so excited to get to work on *Earthrace*, and to have it pulled from under them like this is hard. It's also possible a few will now be laid off. I look around the group. None of it's their fault. They're just doing a fantastic job at building my boat.

Before I know it, work has ceased on *Earthrace* while I continue to scramble for funds. Having failed to raise anything from the very wealthy, we switch our focus to more ordinary people — my old networks of friends from school and work, business people I've been involved with, and a few engineers from the oil industry — anyone I think might be able to help . . . and something very unexpected happens.

People with heaps of money, say more than about a million or so, are very unlikely to loan or donate to *Earthrace*. And in fact a couple were openly hostile that I had the cheek to ask them in the first place. Although, I guess, you don't get wealthy by giving your money away for some guy to build a boat with. But people worth less than a million are prepared to help out. By now I don't really care if the funds are donated or loaned, as long as I get the money to get this beast built. Through this drive I raise a couple of hundred thousand dollars, normally in the form of loans or donations for $10,000 to $20,000.

As soon as the funds start arriving, construction restarts. I'm going through the budgets from Craig, and it seems we're only needing another half million to complete the build. Which sounds like a lot of money, but when you consider it's a three million dollar boat, half a million isn't that much. It's a big asset sitting there. Maybe a finance company will lend me money, using the boat as security.

Tim Costar

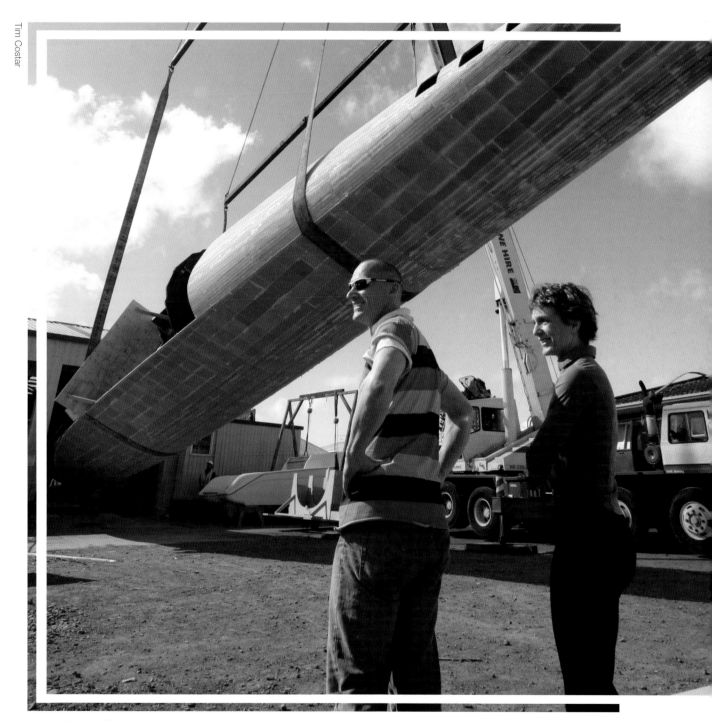

The hull being flipped upside down. Here it has carbon on the inside but none on the outside. Sharyn was upset this photo made her bum look big. Yeah right.

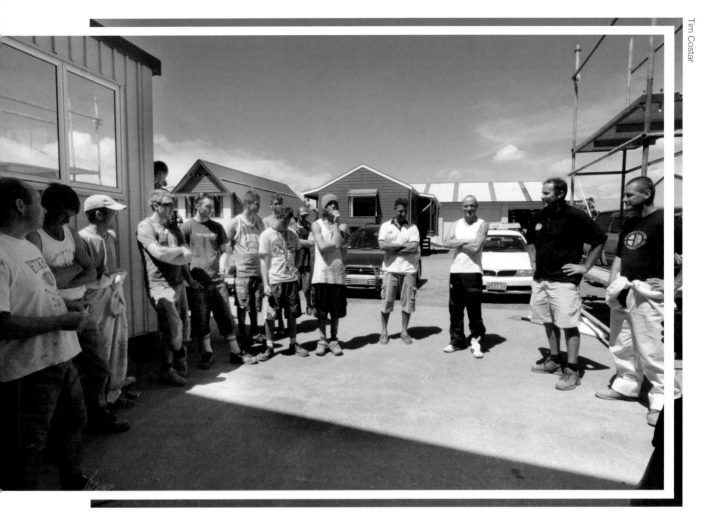

Tim Costar

All smiles but not for long. This is moments before I tell the lads we have to stop construction because we've run out of money. Everyone was gutted.

One company that seems a logical fit is Marac Finance. They have a guy dedicated to marine finance, and after a couple of positive meetings, I'm pretty confident they'll loan me somewhere between $300k and $500k. After chasing them for a couple of weeks we get back a short email declining us because we don't meet their criteria. I spend the next month chasing every other finance company around New Zealand, but gradually give up hope of signing any of them. Construction stops for a second time, and again word goes out that *Earthrace* is doomed.

In one last-ditch attempt to get some funds, I arrange a series of meetings on both the east and west coasts of North America. Ryan is coming with me, the intention being to film the trip, and having a cameraman in meetings would help lend credibility to our claim of making a TV series.

'You can't fly with this,' the airline attendant says to Ryan at Auckland Airport on our way out. 'The photograph is damaged,' and she hands his passport back to him, pointing out the damaged area. We argue the case, but to no avail, so I fly out alone, with Ryan arriving a few days later.

Within the biodiesel community in North America, there is a growing awareness about *Earthrace*, and it allows us to minimise costs by support from locals. Agrifuels loan us a diesel car, and biodiesel companies are all too willing to give us free fuel. We're also staying with a number of different volunteers who have registered on our website. Our only real cost for the trip now is airfares.

We meet with West Coast Reduction in Vancouver and they immediately offer both funds and biodiesel. After that we get some small donations down the west coast, but nothing substantial. The highlight, though, is Willie Nelson, who offers to write us a song. In fact we never did get the song out of him, but it sure gave us a good feeling having the offer made.

The west coast tour in the end is OK, but the east coast trip is just weird. I'd been emailing a young guy called Joseph in New York, who was involved in a project developing a hydrogen-fuelled boat. When he found out what we were up to he immediately started helping us, and he did manage to get us into some good meetings in New York. 'You can also stay at our place,' he offers, which is really appealing, as he lives in the heart of Manhattan.

'Here's home,' he says as we wander into a swanky apartment on the thirty-second floor, 'and this is my mom.' She immediately starts doting on us and making a fuss about things, and pretty soon things are strained. In New Zealand we're so used to having people stay at our house that it's no big deal. And in fact many people in the States we'd stayed with were cool about it. But with Joseph's mum, well, it just seems awkward.

The next day his mother offers to put us up at a local hotel. We pack up our stuff and trundle along to the four-star hotel she's arranged, happy not to be paying the bill in such a luxurious place. A few hours later Joseph calls. 'Umm. Mom doesn't think we should have to pay for your hotel, so we'd like you to pay your own way from here.' It's fair enough really, although there's no way we can afford a place like this. So we pack up our gear for a second time, and wander down to a youth hostel in Harlem, which is way cheaper, and much closer to what we're used to anyway.

Over the following few days we have meetings with several blue chip companies, including American Express, Verizon and UPS. It's like Groundhog Day, though, as they all comment that it's an amazing project, but decline to get involved in any capacity.

Our final meeting is in Richmond, a few hours south of New York. We catch an overnight train down, which saves us one more night's accommodation. By now our funds are getting very low. 'I've only got fifty bucks left,' Ryan says as we wander out of our final, and unsuccessful, meeting. 'How much you got?'

I fossick through my wallet, which is full of receipts, and little in the way of money. 'About forty bucks and my Visa is already dead.'

## 'Do you reckon we're goners Pete?' This trip feels like our last throw of the dice

We sit down on a stoop and look out over the beautiful river that runs through town. It's a magnificent hot day and there are people out enjoying the sun. Somehow our situation doesn't seem so bad, despite being rejected again.

'Do you reckon we're goners Pete?' Ryan finally says, conscious that this trip feels like our last throw of the dice.

I think about this for a while. We have an amazing-looking boat, albeit only half built, and an increasingly loyal group of supporters and volunteers. What we lack is money, and an ability to sell sponsorship or raise funds. If *Earthrace* gets thrown out of the yard, though, which is possible now that construction has stopped, it'll turn into a white elephant with grass growing in it, and we'll never get anyone to support us. But we've made it this far, and somehow I just think we'll continue to get by.

'Do you fancy a swim?' I say, changing the subject. We run across the bridge, down to the river and jump in. The water is brown and murky, but we hardly notice. There's a small knoll sticking out in the river, so we start doing bombs off it. 'Man, it's just like being back in Wanganui,' Ryan exclaims as he scrambles back up the bank. A local policeman comes wandering down, cussing us for swimming in such a polluted waterway.

'But we're from New Zealand bro!' Ryan yells out, as he leaps off the knoll.

We put the rest of our funds into a couple of Greyhound bus tickets back to New York, arriving there around midnight. We're anticipating a long night in the open, but Ryan manages to strike up a conversation with a young woman. 'So where do you live?' he enquires early in the piece.

'Just a few blocks that way,' she says, pointing down one of the side roads. Ryan and I exchange knowing glances. He tells her about *Earthrace* and what we're doing, and finally poses the question, 'Would it be cool if we slept at your place?' She looks surprised at the question and hesitates. 'We're both toilet trained,' I add, 'and Ryan will cook your breakfast.' She finally agrees, and we head off to her minuscule apartment.

In fact the apartment is so small that all three of us end up in her room, me on the floor, with Ryan and Angie sharing the single bed.

We board our flight back to Auckland with two dollars between us. It's a long flight, and I spend most of it wondering where to go to from here. Ryan keeps chipping in ideas, and I'm starting to think he's a lot more useful than I'd originally thought. He was initially on board just to film, but he's getting involved in everything these days. He's unafraid of hard work, manages to get stuff done — and pulling that chick last night: that was impressive.

It's Friday evening when I finally arrive home, and there's an amazing email waiting from South Canterbury Finance. They are prepared to loan us $350,000 at cost, as long as we can raise the other $150,000 necessary to complete construction. I have the usual spaghetti bolognaise and rum and coke ready for Sharyn when she arrives home. She's lounging back on the new polka-dot beanbag that Danielle, my eldest daughter, had scrounged from an inorganic pile down the road. 'I've got good news,' I say, and I tell her about the money from South Canterbury. We then start talking about the other 150 grand.

'We could always sell the forestry block,' I offer hesitantly, passing the glass back to Sharyn. 'That'll give us the full half mill to complete construction.' She has that worried look on her face, like I'm throwing everything away. Not that long ago we had a tiny mortgage, and lots of assets, whereas now all we have left is a forestry block. There's a long silence, while she thinks about it.

'You'd better get that boat launched,' she finally says with a slight smile crossing her face. 'And you'd better get that darn record as well.'

She's an amazing lady, I think. I love her for many reasons, but what she's

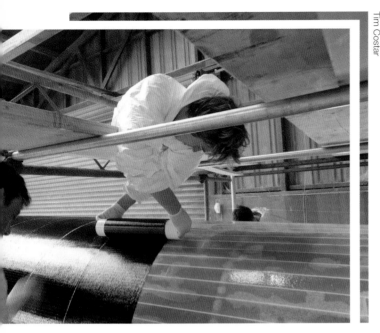

Mike and Jesse applying carbon to the outside hull.

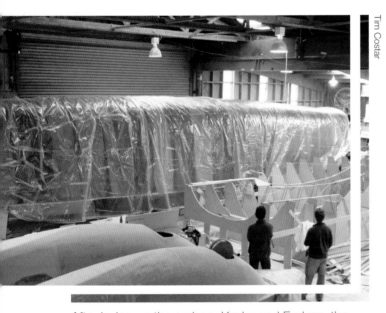

After laying up the carbon, Kevlar and E-glass, the hull is wrapped in peel ply, cloth then a giant plastic bag, and this is all placed under vacuum. It sucks out excess resins, making the hull as light as possible.

just agreed to is way more than any husband could reasonably expect. I finish the rum and get up to pour a new one. I come back and lie down next to her, handing her the glass. 'You're an amazing lady and I love you.'

'I love you too,' she replies. 'Here's to *Earthrace*.'

The forest block is sold, the South Canterbury Finance money comes through, and we're suddenly back in business. Calibre Boats crack into construction, and things are roaring along again. There's also something else starting to happen. *Earthrace* is gaining in credibility, as the boat starts to actually look like a boat rather than a pile of disconnected pieces. We have a web camera following construction, and it's getting a huge and increasing number of hits, as people start to track progress.

'It feels like things are falling into place,' Ryan says to me as we're setting up to film at the yard. It's nearly midnight, and the boat builders are about to start laminating the main hull in one big session. 'Once we start, we must keep going until it's all finished,' Craig says to the lads. 'There are four layers to go on, starting with three carbon, then one Kevlar, and finally one E-glass.' He starts delegating jobs among the team. There are also a few volunteers along, running around with buckets and making themselves useful.

The team finally winds up around six the following afternoon. The laminated hull has been wrapped in a giant plastic bag, which is placed under a vacuum. 'This will help push all the layers together,' Tony is explaining to the camera, 'and it also draws out any excess resins to keep the hull light.' He's been a revelation on camera, young Tony. Craig always has that 'deer in the headlights' look as soon as the camera starts rolling. Tony, on the other hand, just talks like he always does, and it comes across very naturally. He's also quite photogenic in a gnarly kind of way.

With so much progress being made on the boat, we switch our attention to fuel for the race. The trickiest sections are the small Pacific islands that currently have no biodiesel production, and I'm wondering if it'd be possible to set up mini biodiesel plants there to make our fuel along the way. One of the great things about biodiesel is there are so many different sources that can be used. Countries can just use crops or materials most suited to their conditions. In New Zealand, five per cent of our transport fuels can be derived purely from tallow (animal fat) that we process already. Tropical islands can use coconut oil. Africa and the Middle East can use oil from the seeds of the jatropha shrub. Europe and North America already have substantial areas dedicated to canola and soy bean, all of which make great biodiesel. In fact there are over 350 different crops that can be used, covering all continents of the globe.

Ryan and I talked a while back about filming a road trip around new Zealand, where we'd have a mobile biodiesel plant behind a biodiesel car, and we'd circumnavigate the country making our own fuel along the way. We'd start by using butter in Morrinsville, beef fat in Taranaki, used cooking oil in Wellington, olive oil in Nelson, possum fat in Southland, canola oil in Canterbury, sheep fat in Hastings, fish oil in Whakatane, and avocado oil in Northland, which would get us back to Auckland. We would then scrag some fat guy wandering out

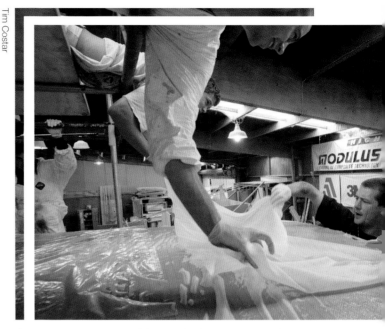

Tim Costar

Tony and the lads applying peel ply to the outside.

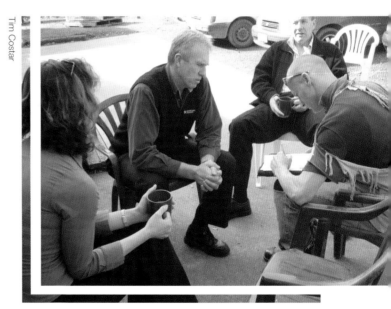

Tim Costar

Sharyn, Barry Woolsey, Steve Wilkinson and myself, signing the loan documents with Auckland Finance. I wore my best jersey for the occasion.

of McDonald's, talk him into undergoing liposuction, and use his fat for the final batch, which would get us back to the Waikato.

In the end TVNZ and TV3 turned us down, but we decide to just do the final bit and run a news item on it anyway. 'I'd like to undergo liposuction,' I say to Dr Rees, one of New Zealand's top plastic surgeons. He frowns at me, no doubt wondering where he's expected to get the fat from. 'And I'd like to keep the fat you remove.' His frown turns to a puzzled look.

'You're not really a suitable candidate for such surgery,' he says, adding, 'I'd be lucky to extract 100 millilitres from your skinny frame.' I explain to him about *Earthrace*, how we're promoting biodiesel, and the many sources it can be made from. After much discussion and cajoling, he agrees to do the surgery, donating his time.

A couple of weeks later and I'm in my gruts lying on his operating table. It had seemed like a bit of a laugh when we teed this up, but now I'm having second thoughts, as the nurse lines up the scalpel, syringes and tools. 'This is the area we're after here,' Dr Rees says, as he draws a dotted line around the base of my back. The nurse squirts a little syringe in the air and hands it to Dr Rees. I feel a few jabs around my back as he injects local anaesthetic. Next comes the scalpel as he cuts two small incisions on either side of my spine.

## I look over my shoulder, expecting a hypodermic-like needle, but it resembles more a giant knitting needle

'This is the needle we'll remove the fat with,' Dr Rees says, as the nurse hands something to him.

I look over my shoulder, expecting a hypodermic-like needle, but it resembles more a giant knitting needle. It's connected by a plastic tube to a small vacuum pump that is humming away merrily. As the needle is pushed into the incision, the vacuum pump changes tone and the first few little bits of fat and flesh start dancing up the tube. It's actually a horrid situation, lying there on the table and hearing part of you getting sucked away. It also surprises me how much force is needed to push the needle along in the narrow fat cavity between skin and flesh. The knitting needle and vacuum pump get swapped for an enormous syringe, and he finishes the job.

'That's all we'll get from you,' Dr Rees says with a satisfied look on his face. He holds up a small container of pinkish fluid.

'It looks like Butter Chicken,' Ryan exclaims, as he and Tim line up some shots of the fat.

'Check this out!' I say to Danielle and Alycia that night at home, proudly holding up the 100-millilitre container of fat. It has separated into three distinct layers — blood on the bottom, flesh in the middle, and fat on top. 'Can I take it to school?' Alycia wants to know. Danielle meanwhile is more interested in the scars, although they're just two tiny incision marks. 'Is that it?' Danielle asks disappointedly after I've removed the plasters.

A surgeon in Wellington sends us around 10 litres of fat, which was from two patients, and our kitchen is turned into a mini-biodiesel plant. Solid human fat is dumped into our big mussel pot, and heated up to eliminate any moisture. The solid yellowy mass turns into a light brown liquid, and we finally add my contribution. It splatters for a few seconds then a few little chunks sit there bubbling away on the surface. 'Hey, it's deep-fried Bethune,' I say excitedly to the camera.

There's actually a slightly weird feeling about all this. Cooking up people's fat in your kitchen just doesn't seem quite right. 'Check out this biodiesel,' I exclaim proudly, as Sharyn arrives home from work. From the initial 10 litres of human fat, we've made about seven litres of biodiesel, and the rest is mostly glycerine, which we throw on the compost heap. Not that seven litres would last long on *Earthrace* with 1080 horsepower grunting away, but it is the first biodiesel ever made from human fat.

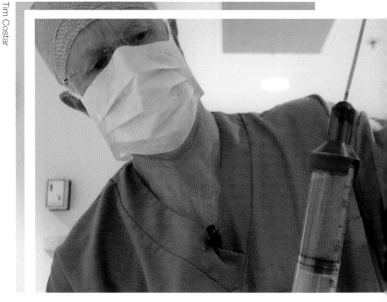

Dr Martin Rees with a syringe full of my fat. He managed to squeeze out 100 ml.

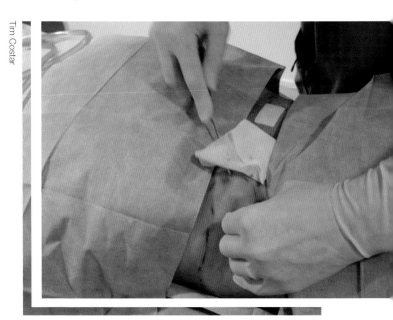

The fat is removed from the base of my back. It was at this time that I started to think what a stupid idea it was. The operation was certainly more brutal than I'd expected.

The launch deadline becomes December 2005, and Craig is initially optimistic about making it. If we can get the boat in the water by then, we'll be able to run a promotional tour around New Zealand between January and March, when everyone is hanging out at the beaches. We'd make some money, raise the profile of biofuels, and get the sea trials sorted, before heading over to North America. Things then started to go astray, however.

The spars are long legs that join in the central hull to the sponsons or outriggers. These are probably the most important structure in the whole boat, and certainly the most expensive. Their shape must be exactly right, but they are a complex curve. The method we devised for making them was to have Greenmount Manufacturing in South Auckland CNC machine polystyrene in small parts that, when assembled, would make up the inside structure. We would then laminate carbon, all 66 layers of it, to the outside of the polystyrene.

The lads at Calibre Boats start laminating but it's a mountain more

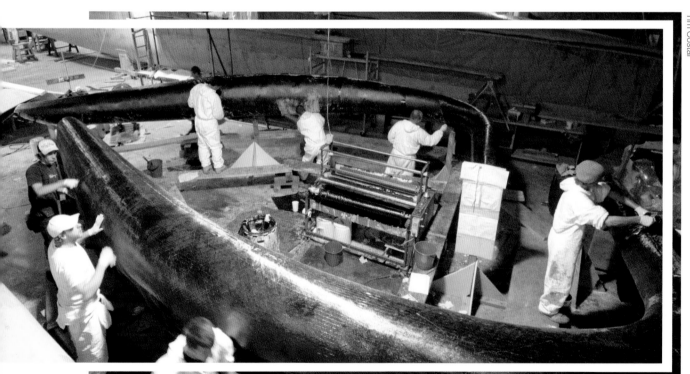

Tim Costar

The ant hive. A late night for everyone as we try and catch up on the spars (in the foreground).

work than they had ever anticipated. 'The trouble is we're only getting a few layers done each day,' Craig explains to me one afternoon, 'and it's just slowed everything right down.' It's become clear that the spars could potentially delay our launch. 'How about we do a few late nights?' I suggest, 'maybe put on a few beers afterwards?'.

'It'll take more than a few beers to get these guys working late. Now that it's warming up, they're all out fishing in the evenings.'

'What about we get a stripper along?' I suggest.

Craig nods his head slowly and smiles. 'Yeah that'll work.'

The night arrives and almost every boat builder in West Auckland turns up to help. We make a huge amount of progress on both spars and the deck. We also get to work on the floor soles, which have composite made from hemp. BMW and Mercedes already use hemp in their composite floor pans, and because it is renewable, it fits with the philosophy of Earthrace.

'Can we smoke it?' Tony says, as he's watching us lay up the first layer.

'Yeah, but you'd need a joint the size of a baseball bat to get a high out of it,' I reply.

# 'Can we smoke it?' Tony says, as he's watching us lay up the first layer

At 2am we're cleaning up when 'Jesse' arrives. 'Where do ya want me to do it?' she says, taking her coat off to reveal a sexy nurse's uniform.

The yard goes quiet as all the lads sneak a look at her while pretending to finish up.

She sets a CD up in my car stereo then lays a blanket down in the middle of the yard. The lads all huddle around in a circle drooling. The stereo is cranked up, and Jesse proceeds to get her gear off, spanking a few cheering boat builders along the way.

The euphoria of the night soon evaporates when the next invoice comes in from Calibre Boats. The half million raised a few months back is all but gone, and *Earthrace* looks far from being launched. 'How can you guys be so far out on your budgets?' I ask Craig angrily.

Craig explains that both carbon and labour were underestimated on the spars. Unfortunately, they carry no liability for this, so it's Earthrace that has to somehow come up with the additional money.

'So how much more do we need?'

'We think a couple of hundred grand will see it launched,' Craig replies, barely looking at me.

So I head off on another scrounge for money. Our house is revalued upwards, allowing Sharyn and me to increase our mortgage by another $50k. South Canterbury Finance increases our loan by another hundred grand, and a few more mates agree to chip in. It seems like these sources have now dried up with this last effort, though.

Much of the work now being done is relatively unskilled, and so we ramp up the volunteer workforce to help out. Friends, family and volunteers start turning up in increasing numbers. Kids from Massey High School in West Auckland and Tangaroa College in Otara also start arriving. Most weeknights see between four and six people helping out, while at weekends it's up to 10 people. Danielle and Alycia even help with the sanding, while Sharyn makes lunches and dinners.

The good thing with this labour is it's free, and it has an ever-increasing number of people taking ownership of the project.

Despite all this, two weeks before Christmas and the 250 grand is all gone, with *Earthrace* remaining a long way from launch. Then, on Monday, construction grinds to a halt.

'As of this morning we have ceased work on *Earthrace*, pending payment in full of all outstanding invoices,' Craig's email had said. It's funny how people will say things in email that they don't want to say to your face. The invoice arrived only a week ago, and the reason I can't pay it is because the project is over budget.

This has become my biggest issue with Calibre Boats. The lads there are doing an awesome job in building an amazing vessel, but we have real budgeting issues. Unfortunately, it is Earthrace that has to continually keep coming up with new funds. The relationship between Earthrace and Calibre Boats is now very strained. I'm continually pissed off because they keep going so far over budget, and Craig is upset because I perpetually owe him money.

Again I ask Craig how much more money it will take to get *Earthrace* launched.

'One hundred and thirty grand. Plus the forty you still owe us,' he replies bluntly, passing an A4 page across the table at me. This is turning into a debacle, I think, eyeing up the fat column of numbers he's written down

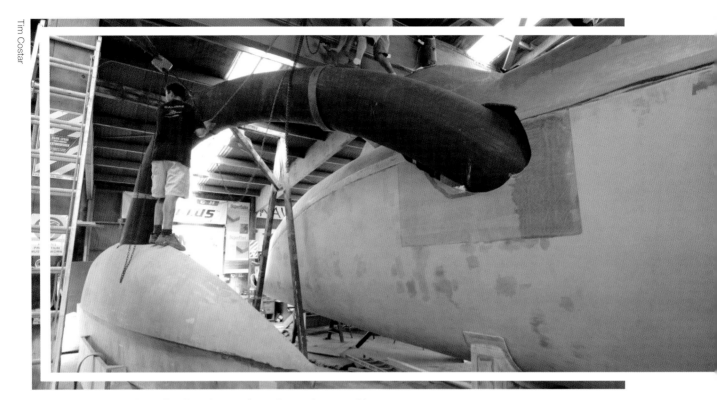

Tim Costar

Craig Ross and Mike adjusting the starboard spar into position.

the side — and so much for being in the water before Christmas.

It's become the lowest point of the entire project. Instead of celebrating a successful launch and touring around the country, I'm left scrambling for further funds, but no idea where they'll come from. I phone around the usual suspects trying to raise some quick cash, but I've squeezed all I can from people who have already been overly generous to me. I'm sick of budgets, and sick of being let down. 'Go on television mate,' Steve had said to me. 'Just say you need some help to get over this final hurdle. The boat is looking amazing now and someone will step up to the plate.'

So in a desperate last bid, I go on TV. 'Just do what you gotta do,' Sharyn encourages me as I head out early in the morning for filming. It's a very soul-searching time, fronting up on national television and pleading for help. It feels like we're a failure for having to do this. TVNZ have us live on their breakfast show, plus an item on the evening news, and TV3 have us on their evening news. 'How much do you reckon we'll raise?' Ryan says that night after we'd watched the final item. 'Hopefully, heaps. We got prime time on both channels, and it is just before Christmas when people are feeling generous. In terms of letting New Zealanders know we need some support, we couldn't ask for anything more.'

Well, we raise a single $100 donation which comes through via the website. 'You're kidding,' Steve says when I give him the news. I load the TV items on our website, then head off to Tairua for Christmas with Sharyn and the girls. I'm gutted with the whole thing and need a break.

Three weeks later and I'm back at home. Looking at our situation it isn't that dire. We're only a couple of hundred grand short of building an amazing boat, and with it so close to being finished, it's unlikely now to end up in a paddock with weeds growing in it. We just need a couple of decent sponsors, donations or loans and we'll piece it all together. I don't know where it'll come from, but I know it will come — and it does.

# He fronts up and throws in fifty thousand bucks. Just like that

The first piece of the puzzle is Tom McNicholl from Biodiesel Oils NZ. This company is the only commercial manufacturer of biodiesel in New Zealand, and Tom's already committed to giving us all the biodiesel fuel we need once the boat is launched. He fronts up and throws in fifty thousand bucks. Just like that.

The second piece of the puzzle is a real surprise. 'Do you know who this is?' the voice says over the phone.

The line is crackly and distant, and the accent if anything sounds slightly Arabic, but like he'd gone to a flash English school. I'm going back through all the Arab people I know but can't place him. 'It's Michael Morcos,' he finally tells me. I'd worked with Michael in the oil industry in Scotland, although now he's based in Dubai as a consultant. 'I've been following your website, and I see you're a bit stuck for money. How much do you need?' I hesitate for a moment, doing some sums in my head. 'About a hundred grand kiwi,' I reply, not really knowing what sort of money Michael has available. There's a long silence. 'Give me your bank account number and swift code and I'll transfer it tomorrow.'

How cool was that? A guy I haven't seen in 10 years just fronted up with $100k after one phone call. And it's not like he and his wife Corinna are

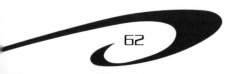

super-wealthy. So there it was: the final funds to get *Earthrace* in the water came from on old mate in Dubai, and a very generous Tom McNicholl in New Zealand. It pays to have faith.

Within 30 seconds I'm back on the phone to Calibre Boats demanding they get right back onto *Earthrace*. Construction restarts for the third time, and my fingers are crossed we'll see it through until launching. There is a mountain of hardware, most of it still racked up at our house, waiting to be installed, so a team of volunteers starts on that. In fact we have so many volunteers turning up now that John Allen takes over managing them all. Ryan and Tim get to work on the launch, now just a month or so away.

Several sponsors, for various reasons, start to back away from previous arrangements. One sponsor tell us at the last minute they'll be unable to complete the job. 'We just don't have the manpower to help you right now,'

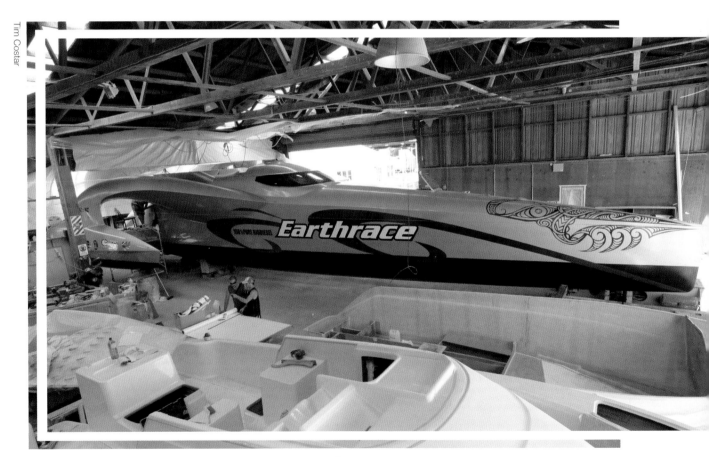

Tim Costar

Earthrace just after the signwriting was finished. Wicked!

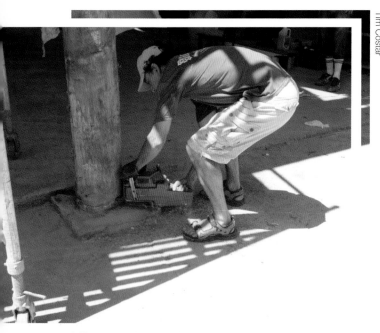

Mike removing a pole that supports the roof. We had to remove this to squeeze *Earthrace* out of the shed.

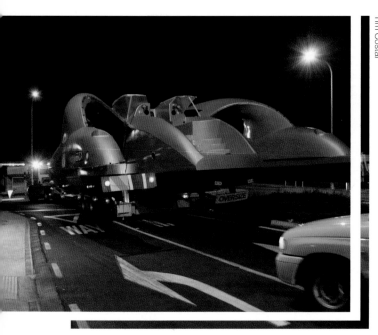

Big boat coming through. We had to pull out lots of road signs to fit through some of the intersections.

one sponsor tells me over the phone. By now, though, it is way too late to get it sponsored elsewhere, so the only option is to contract another company. Considering the number of companies who have sponsored us, the number who haven't been able to assist are few and far between.

Ameron provides a great metallic silver paint, and once this is applied, Rocket Signtists get to work on the graphics. From the start I've always wanted some Maori designs to make it a strong Kiwi boat. Not just a token koru, but some real staunch stuff. Ryan and I stroll into Moko Ink in Grey Lynn to catch up with old friend Inia Taylor, who was the original tattooist on *Once Were Warriors*. 'Yeah I'll come up with something for ya,' he replies after we explain what we want. What he delivers is amazing. On the horns he puts in two korus coming together, symbolising the environment, and around this the positive and negative change in the environment, depending on our actions. The bow graphic is a taiaha (Maori spear), symbolising strength, power and speed. Then there's a small graphic behind the windscreen representing the crew.

I have been busy scrounging stuff on the day the graphics are laid up, and I don't make it to the yard until four in the afternoon, when they are all but finished. I stand there shocked, admiring what surely must be the coolest-looking boat in the world. *Earthrace* has an effect on people. Most see it and are just stunned. It has such beautiful flowing lines, a wicked metallic silver paint job, aggressive graphics. It takes on animal form in some views and a spaceship feel in others. Well, when I see the boat in virtually its finished state, I well up with pride. Here are two years of my life, and the sacrifices of my family and so many others, and the result is just unbelievably good-looking.

Reflecting on the whole process, it is a combination of good management and good luck that has led to this. I have always believed you take on talented people, make them responsible for their area and trust them. Keep tabs on things, but don't interfere and meddle. Partly, this is because these people invariably know more about their field than I do. Also, we are all stretched so thin that none of us have the time to micro-manage the whole process anyway. So Craig Loomes came up with a stunning hull shape, Inia some wicked graphics, Calibre Boats built the beast, and Rocket Signtists finished it off with some outstanding signwriting. End result: brilliance!

Tony and I walk around *Earthrace*, admiring the work. The lads are getting ready to remove the boat from the shed, and they've all got big smiles on their faces. One of them is working a chainsaw on the structure between two roller doors, and sawdust rains down on us as we skirt around the bow. *Earthrace* is so wide that the structure must be removed, giving us effectively a double roller door in width. I look up at the huge amount of roof that will soon be unsupported in the middle. 'You sure that's strong enough?' I ask Tony.

He shrugs his shoulders. 'Yeah, probably.'

A few hours later and *Earthrace* is eased out into sunlight for the first time. She's loaded onto a truck, ready for the trip to Henderson Creek.

At 3am the following morning several TV crews and photographers tag along as we start our slow drive. *Earthrace* takes up basically the

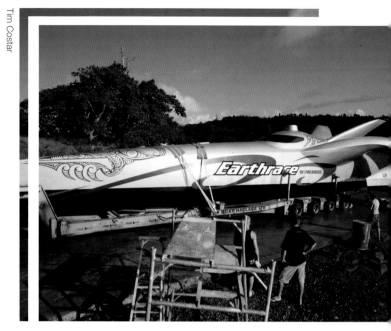

Backing *Earthrace* into Henderson Creek.
Are you sure it'll be deep enough Craig?

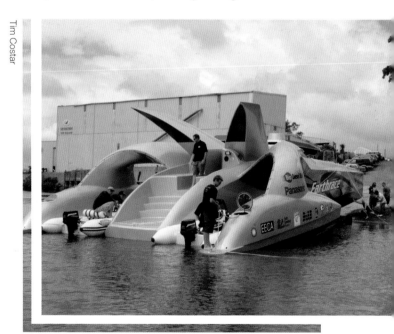

The stern of *Earthrace* just before she floated.
From there we eased her back into Henderson Creek.

entire road width. A couple of us run ahead removing signs and getting cars off the road. Even at this ungodly hour there are lots of vehicles heading in both directions. 'I'll be late for work ya wanker!' one distressed lady yells at me, as I'm coercing her to drive onto the grass verge. 'Oh my God!' she then exclaims, as *Earthrace* looms around the corner. The truck slows for a narrow bridge, the sponsons passing over the railing by just a couple of inches, and then accelerates past the stunned lady's little Corolla.

A few hours later and *Earthrace* is backed into the creek, awaiting the incoming tide. Euro Inflatables have loaned us three little inflatable boats, and we've also got my old boat *Scumbag* to assist. It's 11.23am when she finally lifts off the blocks. A cheer erupts from the hordes watching from the bank, as *Earthrace* floats for the first time.

'Man she sits really high in the water,' Tony comments, as he handles one of the ropes. I look along the hull, and it seems even back around where the engines are, there's only a foot of hull under the water. Being so light, she draws hardly anything. Tim, Ryan and I all scamper aboard, along with a bunch of boat builders, for the slow tow down the harbour into the Auckland Viaduct. We have a launch function to get to, scheduled for the next day.

# Launch function

Two weeks earlier it had seemed like we couldn't even afford a launch function. 'What is my budget for this?' Tim had asked, when we started working on details.

I do a little maths in my head. 'Two thousand bucks.'

Tim frowns. 'And exactly how many people are we expecting?'

I sit there thinking about this for a minute. 'Maybe 100 family members, 200 sponsors and 200 volunteers.'

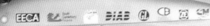
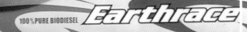

Tim looks down at the floor and shakes his head. 'With only two grand, there's no way we can cater for 500 people. Not unless it's crackers and dip. We all look at each other dejectedly. We've promised so many sponsors and volunteers a great launch piss-up, and to put on a dodgy cheap affair would seem like a real letdown for many of them.

John suddenly sits bolt upright. 'Hey, I know,' he says, a sly smile on his face. 'Let's see who can pull the most fluff out of their belly button.' We all look at him bewildered, and I'm wondering if he's on drugs. John is insistent, so eventually Ryan reaches down into his belly button and pulls out a bit of fluff the size of a matchstick head. He rolls it between his fingers into a ball then flicks it onto the table. 'Oh not bad,' John encourages. I have a go, and almost double Ryan's effort.

# 'Actually, John, I think it's just a reflection of your general lack of hygiene'

Tim then has a crack, his fingers emerging with a ball the size of a small raisin. John then reaches under his shirt. His hand emerges slowly, and unbelievably, in it is a ball of fluff the size of a large marble! He rolls it over a few times between his hands then throws it in the air and it floats down on the table, dwarfing our little samples. 'I win,' he declares triumphantly.

'Actually, John, I think it's just a reflection of your general lack of hygiene,' Ryan suggests, as he pokes the ball of fluff with a pencil. The fluff looks suspicious, though — just a little too fluffy and perfect. John holds his hand up in the air. 'The truth is it's actually the remnants out of my clothes dryer.' He's an interesting character. Who would be mad enough to even think up a game like that, let alone set it up with some fluff out of their clothes dryer?

'John might be the champion tummy fluffer, but it doesn't help us put on a launch function.' I'm keen to steer things back to the launch. There's a long silence between us, as we stare down at the balls of fluff on the table.

'Why don't we just do what we always do?' John suggests. The rest of us sit there wondering what that is. 'We'll just scrounge stuff. Look how much free stuff we got on the boat; we just need to do the same for the launch function. All we really need is some food and some grog.' Actually there is loads more than just that, but food and booze would be a good start.

So we start hitting up companies. 'We'd like two hundred dozen beer for the launch function of *Earthrace*,' I say to the marketing manager of Lion Breweries, and I'm getting into my spiel, when he suggests I go through the usual liquor outlets.

'But we'd like you to sponsor it.'

There's a long pause on the end of the line. 'And why would we do that?' he says, obviously used to getting people phoning up wanting free piss.

'Well, we'll use a bottle of Speight's to christen the boat instead of champagne, and this will screen on *Campbell Live*. In our TV series we'll include footage of the boat builders all drinking Speight's beer. And I'll give you a ride aboard *Earthrace* once we start sea trials.'

There's another long pause. 'How much beer exactly are you looking for?'

'Oh, only two hundred . . . dozen.'

He agrees to the sponsorship, which suddenly galvanises us all into action. Tim is especially good at this, within a few days sorting free wine, Red Bull, bottled water and orange juice.

'How much food do we have?' I ask Tim at our next meeting.

'Um. Some chicken kebabs and sausages.'

'Is that it?'

While the beverages have been easy, food has been surprisingly difficult to scrounge, with the exception of Tegel who were quick to get aboard. I'm mulling this over when my brother Bazza calls from Southland. 'Just got some enormous paua,' he's boasting. 'Would you like me to send up a couple?' I wonder if he could get me a couple of hundred instead?

I explain to Bazza we need as much free food as we can get, and anything wild would be fantastic.

That night he and his son Shaun go spotlighting and shoot a couple of stags near Tuatapere. The following day he meets a local kaumatua and secures a customary fishing permit for 200 toheroa and 250 paua.

'You gotta permit bro?' one of the locals asks Bazza as he's digging around trying to locate the toheroa bed.

Bazza hands the slip of paper over, and continues to dig. 'They're for the *Earthrace* launch function,' he explains.

The local looks suspiciously at Bazza, then a knowing look suddenly crosses his face. 'Dat da funny boat dat runs on fat?' he asks. Bazza nods, and the local smiles.

'No toheroa here bro. They're all over dere,' he says, pointing along the beach. 'I'll go and grab a couple a cuzzies and we'll give ya a hand if ya like.'

Meanwhile some friends caught a couple of marlin off the west coast of Auckland. We never had time for the mussels, scallops and crayfish, but with all the other wild foods, we already had enough for our launch.

Meanwhile Inia Taylor was working in the background for us. He sorted out Tiki Tane from Salmonella Dub to come and DJ for us. Another couple of bands would play for free. We got some flash furniture on loan. We borrowed a big boofy sound system. We just juggled and juggled, stressed to the max, not really knowing how the night would turn out. We just knew that come 6pm on the day, people would start arriving, expecting a great party.

## 'We're running this event tonight whether you like it or not'

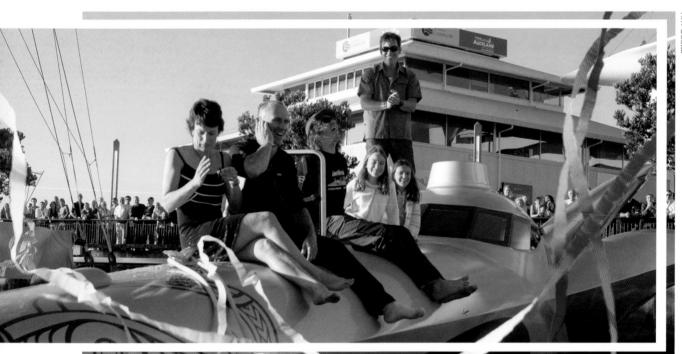

Tim Costar

Sharyn, myself, Ryan, Danielle, Alycia and Tim. We're all laughing because Sharyn has just found out she cut herself smashing the bottle of Speight's on the cleat. Such a sympathetic group.

Suddenly it's D-Day, and the list of things still to do is enormous. Gradually, we start crossing them off. Around lunchtime, though, there's a call from Tim, who sounds desperate. 'We need a resource consent for the marquee, but the council is saying there is no way we can get it today. Without it, we're stuffed.' It's just a standard marquee I'm thinking. Why would they want resource consent for that? I phone up the council department, but the guy is adamant about the consent. I then phone the mayor's office, other city council departments, Heart of Auckland, and a few other people who may have some influence. Finally, I get back to the department head.

'Look. Here's what's going to happen. We're running this event tonight whether you like it or not. The only way you'll stop us is by having a bunch of cops come to close us down. And they probably won't be that keen because there are already a bunch of cops attending. We've got TV3 News and a documentary film crew coming along, and if you actually try to stop us, get prepared for a PR nightmare.' There's silence on the end of the line, before he finally says he'll get back to me, and hangs up.

Half an hour later and the guy calls back. 'While it is most unusual, in this instance we will issue you with a resource consent.' I scramble down to the council, get the permit, and race back to the Viaduct. By now the marquee is almost up.

The fires, however, keep igniting. Some guy called Peter had promised us 15 barbecues and 15 apprentice chefs to do the cooking, but at 5pm he calls to say he hasn't been able to come up with either. Buddha scurries off, and comes back with 15 hired barbecues, just as guests are starting to arrive. We just keep getting problems, and we sort one, only to have another couple thrown at us.

People start arriving and we still have no idea who is doing the cooking. So I just go and grab guests and tell them to get cooking. One of them by chance is Graham Boggs, the CEO of Panasonic, one of our key sponsors. So here he is, with Chris Key, his marketing manager, cooking up toheroa fritters on a barbecue.

We have about 300 people there before I manage to slip away and get changed. When I get back there are more fires to put out. But, gradually, we get on top. It's been the most stressful day in a long, long time. Not just for me, but for all the volunteers. We've hated these last couple of days right up to the event because we knew we were so close to failing. You don't put on

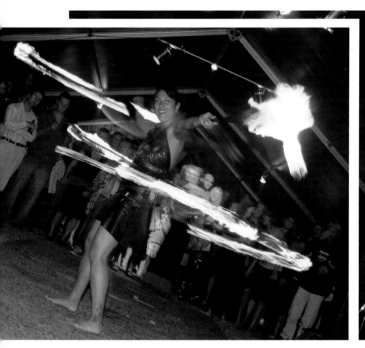

Firedancer doing the business on launch night.

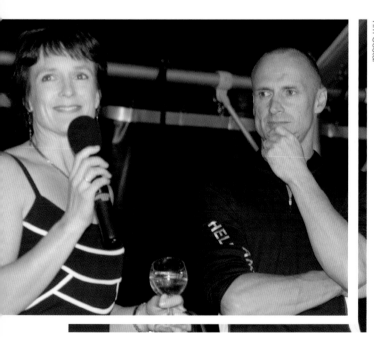

Sharyn saying a few words at the launch function.
One of the proudest days of my life.

an event for 500 people with only two thousand bucks. Or it turns into a disaster.

But like many things on *Earthrace*, we just do our best with what we have, and the result is something special. We thought creatively how to make it happen and we turned it on. In the end it is a wicked night. TV3 film live. As luck would have it the earpiece they give me only starts working seconds before we go live back to the studio. I have a good talk with John Campbell, and Sharyn then smashes a bottle of Speight's beer across the bow cleat of *Earthrace*. Sharyn, Danielle, Alycia, Tim, Ryan and I all sit proudly on the bow.

There are long queues for dinner but heaps of booze to keep everyone happy. The atmosphere is cool, and despite me and all the team being stressed, the night rocks. Inia Taylor brings along a fire dancer. Tiki Tane spins the discs. The bands play. Alcohol keeps flowing. We have a charity auction of various things and raise about $30,000. My bro Bazza arrives up from Southland.

All day I've been trying to get my speech ready but with all those fires, I never get the chance. So when it comes my time to talk, I just stand up and tell everyone about the journey Sharyn, the team and I have taken, and how we haven't done it alone. There is a mountain of people there who have all helped us piece this together. When I get to thanking Sharyn, I burst into tears as she comes up on stage. Sharyn and I have shared something special on Earthrace, but it is more my dream than hers. She has remained supportive, despite our now dire financial situation. And many people there know what a rock she has been.

One thing I have learned through Earthrace is to talk from the heart. Tell people why things are important to you and what you believe in. Let your emotions show. It allows you to connect with people in a powerful way. Tonight is no different. Most of the guests there walk away knowing how important Earthrace is for Sharyn and me, and that it has been a really tough challenge, not for just us, but for many other people who have bled and bled to make the project happen.

One of the changes that has come about in me is I have stopped really caring what the general public think of me. If they see me cry in public, or read about me pleading poverty, or see my bum on TV getting the fat sucked out of it, I don't really care, as long as it helps Earthrace or the environment in a positive way. The funny thing with this is I believe people actually think more of you when you get in this space.

For the core team of Ryan, John, Tim, Sharyn, Steve and me, the launch function feels like the end of a chapter. We have successfully funded and launched the world's coolest boat, and a difficult part of the journey is now complete. From here we have a new set of challenges. We have to stave off bankruptcy, run a promotional tour, and get to the start line early next year. But at least we have a wicked boat.

# Promotional tour

'How much money do we owe?' John asks me in a concerned voice, as we're setting up for our first sea trial on *Earthrace*. I scan the spreadsheet of creditors listing how much we owe and to whom. Towards the end of the build there were several sponsorships that fell through, plus a number of other items we hadn't counted on paying for. We're also now faced with buying items to assist with or sell through the promotional tour. The biggest of these is a marquee theatre, which is over $50,000. 'I reckon by this weekend, our short-term creditors will be about two hundred grand.'

John raises his eyebrows. 'You know the only way we're going to survive is to run an amazing tour around New Zealand, and hope that truckloads of people will pay to board *Earthrace* — and we need to start the tour soon before we go bust.'

The Cummins Mercruiser engineer comes into the helm. 'Ready to go,' he says enthusiastically. John jumps ashore to handle ropes, while I take the controls. We ease *Earthrace* out of the dock and head out into the Waitemata Harbour, *Earthrace* now under her own power for the first time. Both engines are idling away, producing a nice throaty growl. Gradually, we increase engine speeds, and the noise evolves into a loud hum and then a full-on roar, as we hurtle out towards Rangitoto Island.

A film crew from Australian TV series *Beyond Tomorrow* has joined us, and we zoom backwards and forwards to get their chopper shots recorded. 'Man it's got an amazing ride!' yells Craig Ross, as we come across the first few waves. There's just a slight hint of movement as the waves disappear beneath us.

# I've driven my little fishing boat many times, but it's so different to handling this enormous beast

Eventually we idle back into the Viaduct to dock, buzzing with our first sea trial now successfully completed.

'Bow to starboard!' Ryan yells down at me for the third time. I'm busy trying to turn the bow, but the wind just keeps pushing it back towards the dock. John, who remained on shore, scampers along just in time to stop our bow smashing onto the corner.

I've driven my little fishing boat many times, but it's so different to handling this enormous beast. *Earthrace* is extremely light, especially when low on fuel like she is now, and it has her being pushed around by even the slightest bit of breeze. This doesn't matter in open water, but in enclosed waterways like this it makes docking very tricky.

'We need an experienced skipper to join us,' I say to Ryan and Tim as we're tying off the lines. 'I just know so little about driving big boats.' A week later and a guy named Brett has offered to crew with us. 'He's a super-talented guy,' Ryan enthuses. 'He's been skippering boats for ages, and has a wealth of experience.' We meet him for a beer at a pub in Matakana and he seems OK, so he joins our team for the New Zealand tour, now just days away from starting.

Our first promotion is in Tairua on the Coromandel Peninsula, and we arrive there early to get set up. We're planning to open at 9am, but we don't really know if people will come along or not. Or how many people will come down. What we all do know is that our financial position is precarious, and survival from the debt we're currently encumbered with is dependent on open days like today. We'll charge $5 for people to board *Earthrace*, and we'll sell our T-shirts, posters, caps and DVDs. The local newspaper, along with Coromandel FM, have been plugging our presence, so we're hopeful at least a few people will turn up.

At 8.30am the wharf is dead. Then at 9am, a steady trickle of people starts coming through. A few of them have bought T-shirts and caps, and the odd one a poster they want signed. I get a good spot near the ramp and start talking to the public, gradually losing track of time and where we are. An elderly lady with a bright orange dress waits patiently for her turn to ask a question. 'What is your role with all this?' she asks, almost accusingly, and pointing over at *Earthrace*.

# 'Since this morning, we've just been flat stick, and the queue just keeps getting bigger'

'Um, I'm the skipper,' I reply, not really knowing where this is heading. 'Well, I really admire what you are doing, and I'd like to give you this,' and she hands over a massive carrot cake, explaining that her daughter-in-law had cooked it the previous night for us. Just then Tim comes running up to me. 'Can you believe this?' he says excitedly, pointing at the queue of people, now extending along the wharf and almost past the harbourmaster's office. 'Since ten this morning, we've just been flat stick, and the queue just keeps getting bigger.' I check the time, and surprisingly it's already 3pm. We haven't even had lunch yet. I hand the cake over to Tim, and ask him to dish it out to all the crew and volunteers. The lady looks on happily as Tim scampers off down the wharf with her cake.

It's 7pm before we finally get the last of the people through *Earthrace*

Tim Costar

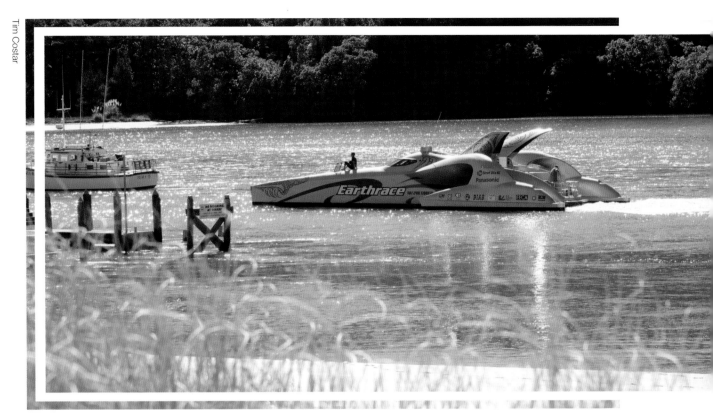

Pulling into the beautiful Whangamata Harbour for Easter Weekend.

and pull away from the wharf. Amazingly, there are over a hundred people there to wave us off, with still more lining the water's edge. As we head around Paku Hill and out towards open water, a small flotilla of boats grows and follows us out, all with kids and families waving and wishing us well. Ryan, Tim, John, Sharyn and I sit on the roof of *Earthrace* and soak up what has been a truly unbelievable day. 'How cool is this?' John says, putting his camera down and leaning back. 'You know Pete. We might just be able to make this promo tour work.' I sit there looking out to the beautiful Alderman Islands, bathed in sunlight from the setting sun, and reflect on the day. We connected with so many people today. People of all ages and demographics, and they all seemed genuinely interested in what we are doing. Regardless of what money we made, the people of Tairua certainly know what biodiesel is now, and hopefully we made an impression on some of them.

Today, in a small way, has vindicated what we've been telling sponsors.

I always believed people would be interested in *Earthrace*, and that media would support us, but the hard part was convincing companies that this was the case. 'It's just a boat. Why will anyone care about it?' a VP-Marketing in the US had said to me some six months ago. For a time there I'd started to wonder if he was right. Maybe people wouldn't really care. Well, after today I reckon they do. While Tairua is a small town, it's still been an enlightening day, and bodes well for the rest of the tour.

The next day we have a similar experience in Whitianga. A downpour around lunchtime reduces the queue for a while, but then the sun comes back out and so do the people. John strides along the dock with a big smile on his face. 'Hey, guess what? Smitty's Sports Bar has offered us free burgers and beer tonight. Oh, and a guy on the dock gave me this,' and John hands over a cheque for 500 bucks.

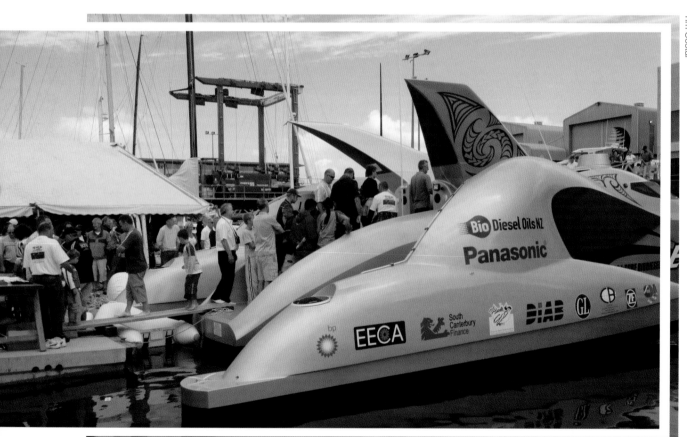

At an open day in Auckland. At times it was like a scrum inside *Earthrace*.

Over the next month, we visit Whangaroa, Russell, Opua, Kerikeri, Whangarei, Auckland, Tauranga, Whangamata and Coromandel with varying degrees of success. It seems as long as we get reasonable media, people will come to see us. It has now brought us to our first long voyage aboard *Earthrace*, from Auckland all the way around the east coast to Gisborne. There's a little bit of trepidation among the crew, as we head off on a windy afternoon for the long haul. 'What's the weather doing?' Brett asks as we cruise towards Colville Channel.

'A storm has been lashing East Cape, but it should have abated by the time we get there. Overall it should be a sweet run.'

The following day, and all that remains of the storm is a rolling three-metre swell. There is also the odd branch and log floating around. 'It might be better if we head further offshore as we work down the coast,' Brett says, as another piece of wood clunks against our carbon hull. We end up 20 miles offshore, and work our way south, with night closing in.

It's 1am when I'm suddenly woken by a thundering crash and the sound of splintering carbon, followed by a series of thuds and shudders. In an instant we're all up, thinking we're about to sink. 'Check the engine room!' I yell to Brett, who is sitting in the helm and looking stunned. Ryan scurries back to the stern to see what we've hit, while I head forward to check for leaks in the bow. There's no water coming in, so we start from the stern looking for damage. 'Check this out,' says Ryan, shining his torch at the port sponson. Shards of black carbon are protruding through yellow Kevlar, and chunks of pink fairing compound are hanging down. The starboard sponson has similar damage, but I consider that neither is about to sink us. Even if we lost the whole sponson, we'd still be able to limp into port.

The loud crash was from the main bow, but to swim around there at night with the large swell rolling in would be dangerous. I think for a minute about how the bow is made. The front two metres are solid carbon, Kevlar and foam, and so the entire tip could be smashed off and we'd still not take on water. The next two metres is a sealed ballast tank, so damage through there would also not sink us. Then the next section, again about two metres in length, is a sealed storage area. So you'd need to smash past at least six metres of bow before we'd have significant water ingress into the main hull. So it is unlikely we're anywhere near sinking.

The following morning we limp into Gisborne at eight knots then sort two cranes from C. R. Taylor to pull *Earthrace* from the water. The bow

79

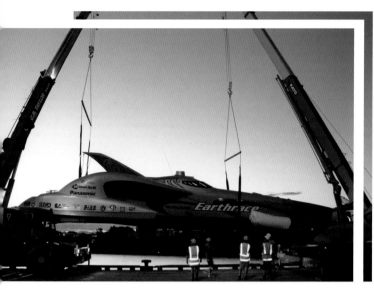

Tim Costar

*Earthrace* being pulled out of the water after we smashed into a log out from Tolaga Bay. The blue sky was not to last long.

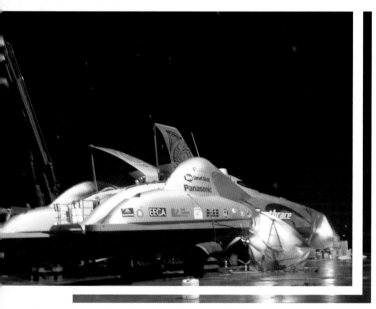

Tim Costar

Repairing the three bows in Gisborne during sleet. The blue tarpaulins were to protect the new composite from rain, while lights are inside to accelerate the hardening process. It was a long and miserable night.

has a large bite out of it where the log initially struck. It looks like the log actually broke in half, because we can see where one piece scraped down the port side and one down the starboard side. The scrape marks can be left for now, but that still leaves all three bows and one rudder to repair. 'There's at least a week's work in all that,' Chris Coppin, the local composites maestro, says on seeing the damage.

'We don't have a week. We have a day,' I say to him, conscious of all the promotional and sponsor obligations we've got lined up.

Chris rolls his eyes then shakes his head. 'There's no way mate. All I can do is my best.'

Two hours later and he's back with a couple of lads and a mountain of gear. As the night rolls on, the weather just gets worse and worse. We sling tarpaulins over the bows, but the rain at times is almost horizontal. Chris continues his sanding, scraping, mixing and cutting, working from one bow to the next in atrocious conditions. Various lights are placed over the repair areas to help in curing the resins, but power keeps cutting out as water gets into the various fittings. Night rolls into day and, amazingly, by early afternoon the following day, Chris and his team have all but finished. I sit there watching them applying the final layer of paint. There's a fantastic work ethic among Kiwis. These guys have worked all night and all day, and they're still just soldiering on to finish the job. We could have been laid up here for almost a week, which would certainly have hurt us badly, but instead we'll be back into the tour with only Gisborne being affected.

*Earthrace* is lowered back into the water and reloaded with fuel and gear. Forty, knot winds greet us as we head out of Gisborne Harbour.

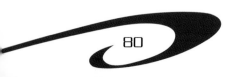

'This will be interesting,' I say to the lads, as we approach Mahia Peninsula. The waves start at only three metres in height, but then build ominously to around six metres, once we're exposed to the southerly storm now whipping up the North Island. It's the first time we've been in really decent waves, and the thing that surprises me is the violence of it all. I had this vision of *Earthrace* slicing through the waves like a hot knife through butter. In reality, it is a brutal exercise, with the boat being pushed and shuddered in all directions as it passes through waves.

I've also noticed that the ride gets better at speed. If you slow right down below 15 knots, the ride is very up and down, more like that of a conventional design. As speed is increased, the piercing increases, and the boat has a flatter trajectory through waves, but there are more jolts and shudders with it.

Everyone by now is in the helm, our emotions a mixture of excitement and fear, as wave after wave comes rollicking over the top of us. Ayla is

Tim Costar

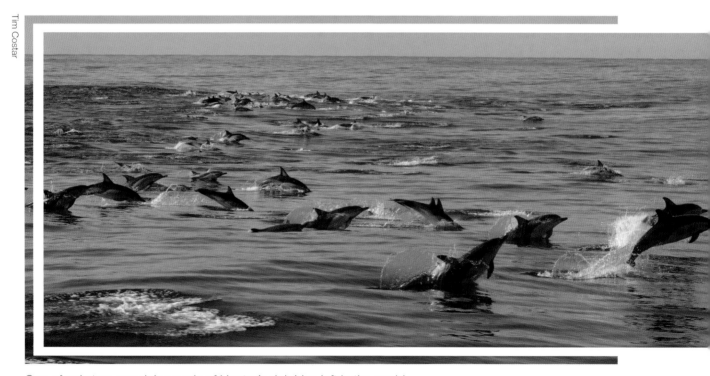

One of only two remaining pods of Hector's dolphins left in the world. We saw both of them on the NZ tour, this one out from Napier, and the second near Dunedin.

yahooing, Ryan is filming, I'm driving, and Buddha (my nephew, who has volunteered for a bit) is throwing up into the chilli bin. We finally reach Napier and make our way behind the Bluewater Motel, which has sponsored us for a few days. It's a very tired and weary crew that amble off *Earthrace*, and into the bar for a beer.

We have a great weekend of promotion in Napier then head down to Wellington. 'Hey, the Don is here for a tour,' John says, as I'm busy organising the docking lines. I look up to see, then Leader of the Opposition, Don Brash and a few of his colleagues, plus a throng of photographers and cameramen all come wandering down. Don graciously allows me to chew his ear for five minutes. 'Do you know that we are the only country in the OECD that doesn't have biofuels available to the public for road transport?' I say, with the cameras all rolling.

# We head down to the boat, and Don suddenly hesitates when he sees the plank he must walk across

'Well, we are working on a policy for biofuels now,' he replies, 'and this will be released in a few months.' I do my best in explaining what we should be doing here in New Zealand.

'For a start, you should make five per cent biodiesel compulsory in all diesel and five per cent ethanol compulsory in all petrol. Simple, really.' One of his minders is taking notes, although I'm not really sure if he's just doing it for show.

We head down to the boat, and Don suddenly hesitates when he sees the plank he must walk across. All the cameras start to roll and click. He gingerly steps across the gap and shuffles along the plank. We had hoped to get a decent news item about biofuels, and promoting the fact that *Earthrace* is open to the public all weekend, but instead it turns into the 'Don walking the plank'. Shots and footage of him are scattered across New Zealand media for days, but it does little to promote what we care about, and perhaps hastens his demise as Leader of the Opposition.

All things considered, though, Don Brash was good enough to come down, so it's a shame we may have inadvertently played this role. Not that I'm particularly enamoured with either the National Party or the government. Despite making a few requests, we've had no assistance from any government department, on a national or local level, with the exception of a $100 donation from Bob Harvey, the Mayor of Waitakere City. Early on when we were really scraping, I visited Tourism New Zealand, who sent me to the overseas trade department, who then referred me on to Jim Anderton. I visited him in Wellington, but he just sent me back to the trade department and Tourism New Zealand. From there we gave up on getting any government support, hoping we'd be able to piece it together without them.

It's a quiet few days in Wellington. With media concentrating on 'Don walking the plank', few people there knew we were open to the public at all. To make matters worse, there's another storm brewing. I return to the boat after talking to a couple of local schools, and the wind is howling. It won't be a pleasant voyage tonight, I think. I look over to where our marquee theatre is; it's sitting precariously close to the edge of the dock, half disassembled, and people running everywhere pulling it to bits.

I rush over to John to see what's going on. 'I was just sitting over here,' he says, 'when a gust of wind hit, and the whole marquee moved about 10 metres, concrete blocks and all. One end collapsed, and then a couple came running out screaming. Then another gust hit and the whole thing teetered on the edge of the dock. I honestly thought it was gone.' I look over to what remains of the marquee. It's just a tangled bunch of frames, with Ryan running around barking orders. It takes another hour before the parts are pulled to bits and loaded safely into the truck, although many of them are

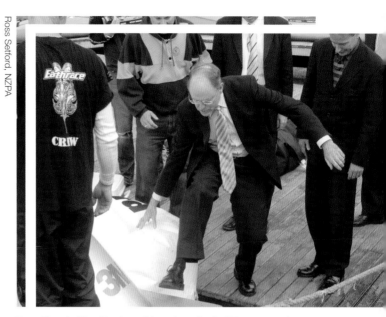

Ross Setford, NZPA

Don Brash (the Don) walking the plank. Photos and footage of this were played over and over in subsequent weeks, as the Don's political career tumbled.

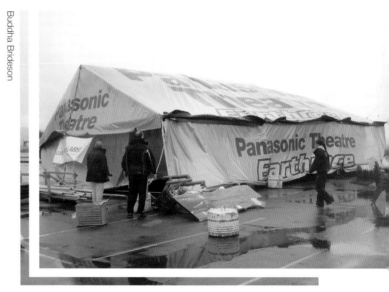

Buddha Brideson

Our Panasonic marquee theatre close to being swept out to sea. It teetered on the edge for several minutes while the crew tried to save it. Note the left-hand side has collapsed.

now bent. 'You know I'm not really so sure about continuing with this marquee,' John says. 'It's just too much hassle.'

In fact the marquee has turned into a white elephant. The idea was to screen the *Earthrace* TV documentary, but people just don't seem inclined to hang around for it. 'I brought my kids to see a boat, not a movie,' a guy had said to me earlier in the day.

'Maybe we should just ship it back to Auckland and sell it,' I say to John, closing the door on the back of the truck. Not my wisest investment, I muse. It cost over fifty grand, we've only used it a few times, and now we're going to sell it, bent poles and all.

# The first big wave picks us up and Ayla yelps in fear, as our bow points precariously down into the wave trough in front of us

We head out from Wellington and into Cook Strait with the winds, according to the radio, now gusting 60 knots, and seas at eight metres. The airport has been closed and the inter-island ferries have stopped operating. The first big waves come smashing over us, and within a few minutes Buddha has joined his chilli bin back in the galley, for what he knows will be a long night. A few of the waves seem much larger, maybe up to 12 metres in height but, surprisingly, *Earthrace* handles them with relative ease. After two hours of slow progress, we do almost a U-turn, to make our run back through Cook Strait towards Nelson. It's the first time we've been in a large following sea, and everyone is anxious.

The first big wave picks us up and Ayla yelps in fear, as our bow points precariously down into the wave trough in front of us. The steering becomes light, the propellers cavitate slightly, and there's a loud whooshing sound as we zoom along, surfing the wave. After a short distance we fall off the back face and slow down. On the next wave I steer it manually, trying to angle *Earthrace* at about 10 degrees to the wave. Amazingly, we just surf on and on. At times it feels like we're about to nose-dive and, at others, like we're about to flip. *Earthrace*, though, just keeps on surfing the wave, zooming along at 25 knots, and with the engines hardly loaded at all. I glance down at our GPS, and see we've been on this wave for over three miles, and still going. Finally, we fall off the back. 'Man, how cool was that?' Ayla says with a hint of relief in her voice.

Craig Loomes has always said *Earthrace* would handle well in a following sea, but over the last few months many people have disagreed. 'It'll pitch pole and you'll be upside down before you know it,' a gnarly old seadog had said to us in Napier. Well, today we handled a big eight-metre following sea, and the boat handled it brilliantly.

We run promotions in Nelson, Christchurch and Timaru, unfortunately skipping Kaikoura because they cannot find us a suitable floating dock. Next we head to Dunedin, where there has been a loyal band of volunteers organising things for us.

That evening, however, after our first open day, we realise that our days with Brett as part of the crew cannot continue and, suffice to say, he is asked to leave. It's a shame really. Brett has been the only guy capable of docking

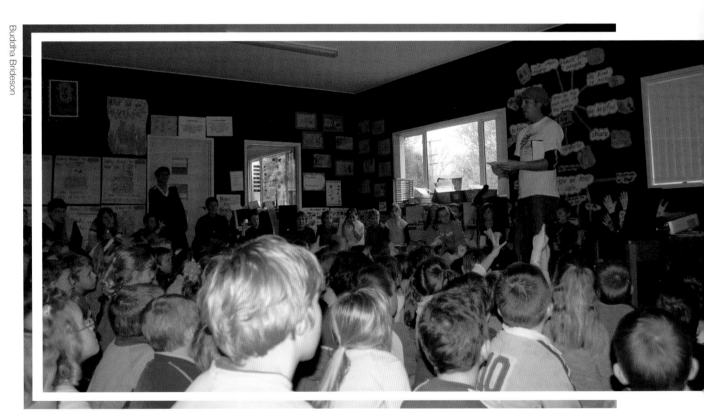

Buddha Brideson

Tim Costar talking at a primary school in Dunedin. The crew got a real kick out of these talks.

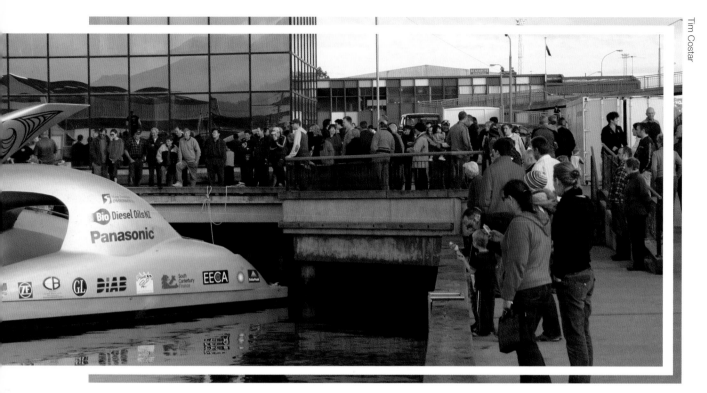

Tim Costar

Open to the public in Dunedin. The dock was chock-a-block with people all weekend.

the boat properly. The few times I've had a go I've gotten into trouble. So from now I'll just have to front up and make it happen. We're also about to head over to the west coast, and having Brett's nautical experience along that rugged coastline would be invaluable. However, Brett hadn't really fitted in. So maybe it's for the best.

'Hey, I know,' says Ryan. 'Instead of moping around here, let's go and watch the Taliband play. They've got a gig just down the road.' We grab our jackets and head out, still smarting from an emotionally charged day. Ryan starts singing one of the Taliband songs as we squeeze into the lift. 'Life is a dinner plate. Do, do, da, do, do, do . . .'

Dunedin turns out to be a record for us, and the boat is filled with people all weekend. It's funny how some cities have embraced us and some haven't. Christchurch a few days earlier had been pretty ordinary, with little in the way of sponsorship, limited media coverage, and few people boarding *Earthrace*. Here we've had various hotels, restaurants and pubs sponsoring us. Several companies came down and helped us set up, loaning us equipment. All the schools welcomed the crew to come along to talk to their classes or assemblies, and local media have been really keen on covering us, one of their radio DJs even wakeboarding behind *Earthrace* to promote us.

We leave Dunedin very satisfied. It almost feels like a new start. I'll get you to drive from here,' I say to Ryan, once we're safely over the bar and heading south. Ryan jumps into the driver's seat and leans back. 'What an amazing few days that was,' he says.

'Of all the places we're going to visit, I reckon it'll be hard to top that.' He leans forward and engages the autopilot. 'Next stop Stewart Island.'

'Hey, check out the view,' says Buddha, scampering into my room and pulling the curtains. I squint from the sudden burst of light, but obligingly lift my head and look out the window. We're in the beautiful old South Sea Hotel in Halfmoon Bay on Stewart Island, and the view is just stunning. Bush-clad hills surround us, and water laps against a gorgeous beach just a few metres from the hotel's front door. I look over towards the wharf and there is *Earthrace*, already with a small crowd of people gathering around her. 'Oh you're giving a talk at the school in half an hour so you'd better get up,' Buddha says, running out of the room, eager to wake up the rest of the troops.

That evening we play the *Earthrace* DVD at the hotel, and there's an amazing turnout, considering the island has only 350 permanent residents. 'Must be half the island here,' John says, eying up the crowd. An old man comes up

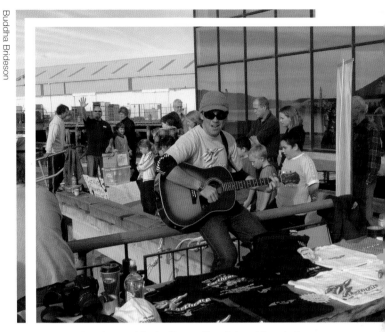

Tim entertains the public in Dunedin. John Allen is in the back waving.

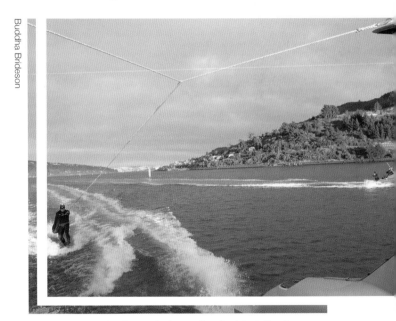

A Dunedin radio DJ wakeboarding behind *Earthrace*. We use the horns as tow points, which help lift the wakeboarder up.

and shakes our hands. 'Was that you docking the boat last night,' he says to me, putting his beer down on the bar.

'Yeah, it was.'

'My grandmother could do a better job,' he says caustically, and he emits a raspy laugh. I look at the old man. His face is wrinkled and weathered from years in the wind and sun, and his hands are rough and worn. Must be a fisherman, I think. The docking *was* a bit ordinary, though. There's a certain rustic charm about the people here which I find endearing. Good, honest, hard-working people who call a spade a spade. Isolation also tends to make them hugely independent and capable as a community.

A middle-aged lady comes up to join us, leaning on the old man and giving him a kiss. She's drinking Jack Daniels and coke, and has had a few more than just the one in her hand by the looks of it. 'You know, there's two

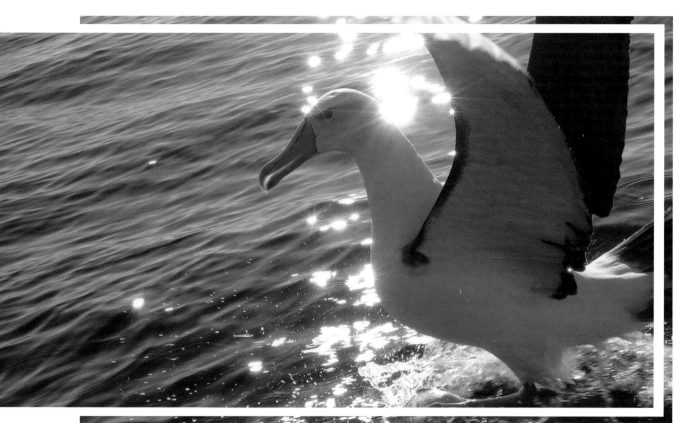

Buddha Brideson

The indignant mollymawk a few minutes after Buddha had caught it. Magnificent birds.

great things have happened on Stewart Island,' she says. 'Billy Connolly came here . . . and now *Earthrace* has also been here.' We toast Stewart Island and *Earthrace*, and a few more locals come over to join us.

It's an early start the following day, but a nice turnout of locals still make it down and see us off. The old man is there, as well as the middle-aged lady with a handful of kids, all waving their arms furiously. The water is dead flat and there's not a cloud in the sky. We travel a few miles, and are just rounding a shallow reef the locals had told me about the night before. I pull the throttles back and put *Earthrace* in neutral. 'What are we doing?' Ryan asks.

'We're going for a fish and a dive.' I grab the dive gear and head outside, while Ryan and Buddha struggle with the anchor.

An hour later and I'm back on deck. My body has got the tired but satisfied feeling I often get after a good dive. I lie back in the sun warming up, while the rest of the crew dangle baits off the back of *Earthrace*. There's a flock of large birds sitting in the water eyeing up the baits. 'What kind of birds are those?' Ryan says, as he's threading a pilchard onto a hook. They're similar to albatross, but a little smaller. 'Mollymawks I think,' says Buddha. A few seconds later and pandemonium breaks loose, as the mollymawks all start squawking. I look over and there is Buddha with a big mollymawk, thrashing its wings angrily, as it tries to race off with Buddha's bait. The reel screeches intermittently as line is pulled off, with Buddha looking on and wondering what to do. Thankfully, the hook eventually pulls out, and the sullen bird sits a distance away glaring at us indignantly.

Buddha gives up the fishing, and decides to fossick through my catch bag instead. Six good crayfish, the largest a bit over two kilos, a bunch of kina and some paua. 'Man, we'll dine like kings tonight,' he says enthusiastically. We're going to stay at my brother's place in Riverton. Bazza has also lined up whitebait and oysters for our banquet — maybe a bit of venison out of the freezer as well.

We run our last two South Island promotions in Riverton and Bluff. Despite the wind and rain, both places are fantastic. Many years ago Peter Blake ran a similar promotional tour around New Zealand with *Ceramco*, his first 'Round the World' yacht. Apparently, Bluff was where he raised the most funds, closely followed by several other southern cities. Well, we've had a similar experience, with Dunedin being tops, and the other cities down south all being awesome.

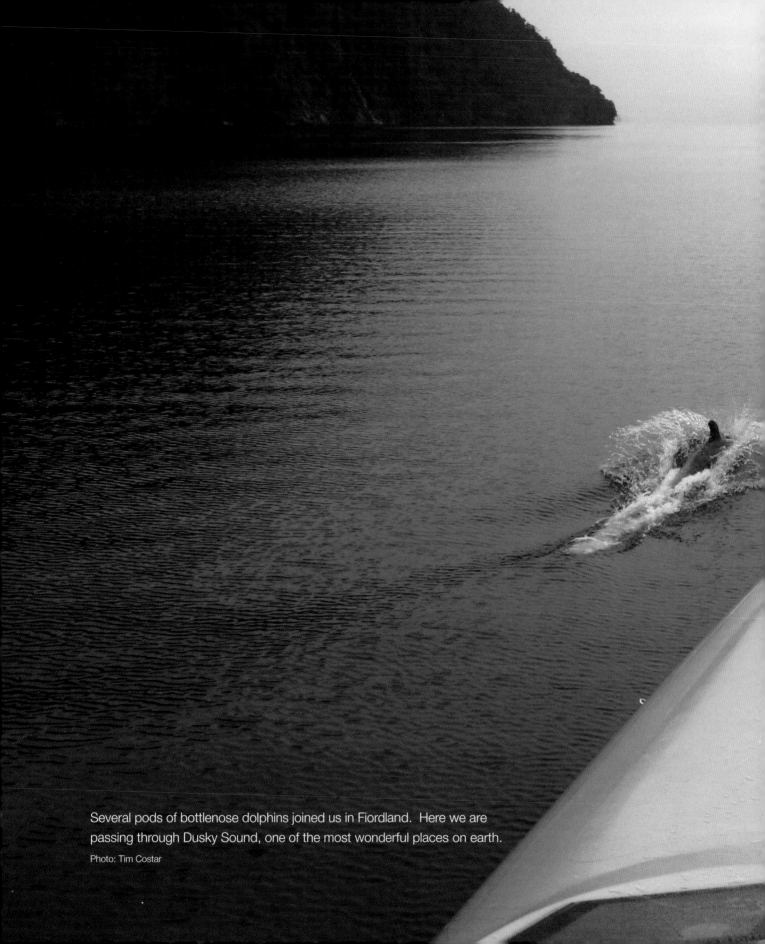

Several pods of bottlenose dolphins joined us in Fiordland. Here we are passing through Dusky Sound, one of the most wonderful places on earth.

Photo: Tim Costar

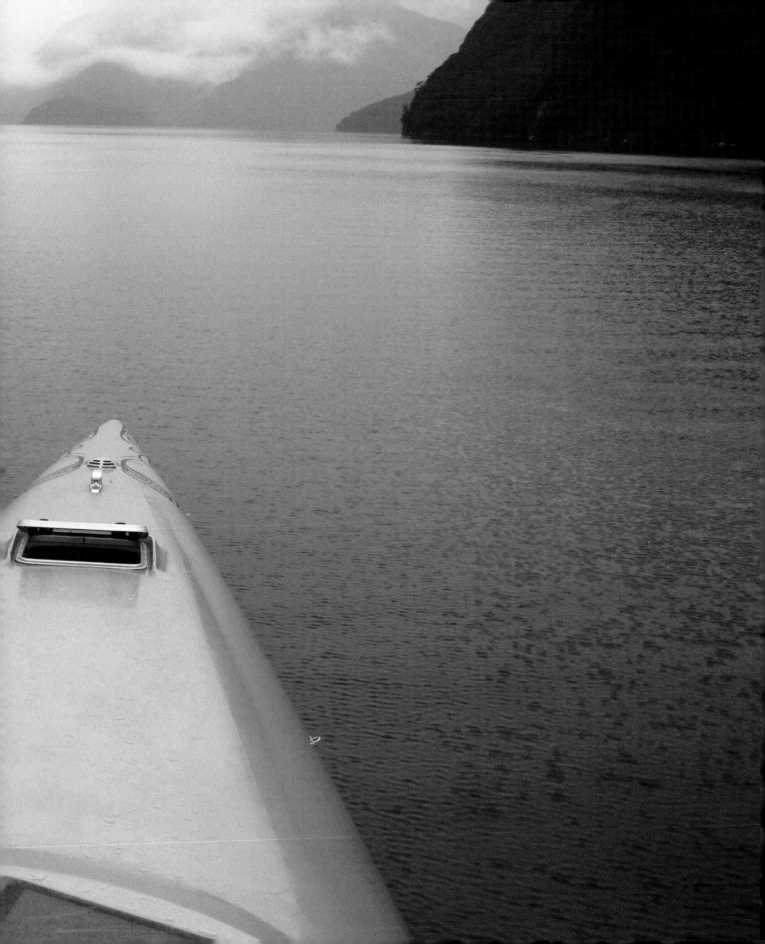

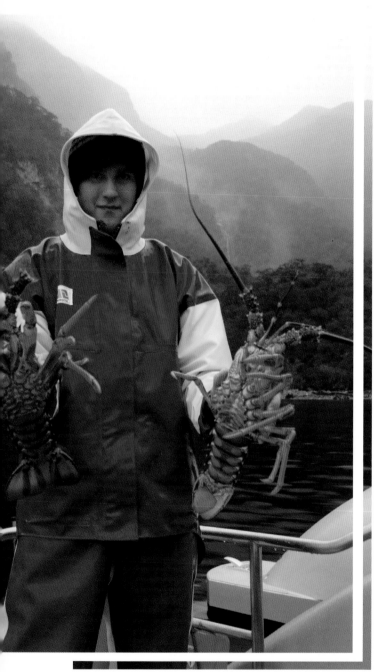
Tim Costar

Torsten Sandmark getting ready to cook up my fat Dusky crayfish. Note the mist in the background. This stayed with us the entire time we were in Fiordland.

From Bluff, we pack up our gear and head off to Fiordland for some adventure. We idle up Dusky Sound through the night, and awake to a dark and brooding overcast day. There's a rugged majesty about Fiordland that is only really appreciated by being here. It is almost completely devoid of human activity, aside from the occasional commercial fisherman. Sheer cliffs rise out of the water on either side, up to snow-clad hills and mountains. Every 500 metres or so a waterfall careers down into the crystal waters.

'Hey, we've got company,' Torsten, our new crew member yells, as a pod of bottlenose dolphins comes bounding towards us. They hang around for ages, searching for the best wake to ride on, and every now and then one athletically leaps out of the water. Ryan, Tim and Buddha sit on the roof working their cameras and enjoying an amazing spectacle. Surprisingly, the dolphins remain with us for over an hour, as we head up to find an anchorage.

It's late afternoon before we finally get the anchor to hold. 'It'll be a dark dive,' Bazza says to me, looking at the mist and clouds surrounding us. He's struggling pulling his wetsuit on, which is a size too small. 'It's my winter condition,' he says, reading my mind as I'm eyeing up his swollen belly. We finally get all kitted up and jump over the side. The fresh water on the surface is bitterly cold, but as we get down it suddenly warms as we enter the salt layer. The boundary between the fresh and salt water also acts as a sound barrier, and it's eerily quiet as we head down towards the dark rocks some 10 metres beneath us. I feel both excitement and foreboding, with the thought of big crayfish being tempered by the gloomy quiet conditions that surround us.

We start on a ledge and work our way around, looking for feelers. Some 10 minutes later and I spot the first crayfish. A good buck around a kilogram, backing into a hole, his feelers dancing backwards and forwards towards me. I grab him and tuck him down into my catch bag. There follows a long section of reef with little in the way of crevices or boulders for crayfish to live in. A big gloomy shadow looms in front of us, as we work our way along and up to a sheer face. Edging closer, I can see the face is covered in deep crevices, all working their way down towards the depths. Crayfish country!

I drift near the first ledge and look along it, almost knowing it'll hold a crayfish or two. Amazingly, though, there are crayfish scattered all along it — at least a dozen of them, all jostling for position as their feelers pick up our vibrations in the water. I pick out the biggest set of feelers, and after a short wrestle, pull out a beautiful two and a half kilo buck. I look down to the next crevice, and it too is chock-full with feelers.

## As we near the point, *Earthrace* comes into view, drifting away from us

A short time later and we've got six great crayfish, so Bazza and I head back to the surface, some 25 metres above us. 'How wicked was that!' says Bazza, pulling off his mask. 'Hey, Pete. Small question: where is the boat?' I look back up to where the boat was anchored and it's gone. Ryan knows to stay right near us, and yet they've disappeared.

'Let's swim down there and have a look,' I say, pointing to the peninsula some 200 metres further south.

As we near the point, *Earthrace* comes into view, drifting away from us. I yell out, and someone suddenly jumps on the roof and starts yelling at us. 'Can you make out what they're saying?' Bazza asks, his hearing impaired from years of shooting rifles. I pull off my wetsuit hood but they're just too far away to make it out. Although I can tell they're excited about something.

'You stay here and hang onto this,' I say to Bazza, handing him the catch bag, and I start swimming toward *Earthrace*.

I make little progress, with the boat drifting away almost as fast as I'm swimming. I then see the guys wrestling with the anchor rope, which is still hanging over the side. Dusky Sound is 500 metres deep here, so there's little chance of it grabbing anything. *Earthrace* is gradually drifting towards the cliffs where the fiord narrows, and I can see the waves crashing against the rocks. What the hell are they doing?

Ryan and Torsten have worried looks on their faces, as I drag myself up onto the transom step and collapse. I'm exhausted from the long swim, but something sure isn't right. 'Our anchor didn't hold, and we're unable to start the engines,' Ryan says quickly. 'The wind just keeps pushing us towards that,' and he points to the cliffs, now just a couple of hundred metres away, and directly in our path.

We hurry into the helm. The ZF alarm is sounding, so I push the 'clear' button, and both engines fire up first time. 'Which button was that?' Ryan says, a real sense of relief in his voice. I explain to him how the ZF system needs to be cleared if the main circuit breakers are switched off. 'Pull the anchor up guys, Bazza will be freezing back there.' We hurry back to pick up Bazza, still bobbing up and down by the peninsula with our bag of fat crays.

We pack up and head off for Milford Sound, where a photo shoot has been organised. It's a gorgeous day in what must be one of the most stunning fiords anywhere in the world. 'What's for dinner?' Ryan asks, as we stop the engines and drift in the middle of the sound.

'Crayfish bro,' replies Tim, as he's busy trying to start our biodiesel cooker. 'In fact it is a crayfish each, so I hope you're hungry.' An hour later and we're all sitting on the roof of *Earthrace*, tucking into an enormous feast of crayfish, paua, blue cod and salad. The mountains around us fade out of view as darkness sets in, and the sky is ablaze with stars. 'I'm stuffed,' Ryan says finally, as he rubs his stomach lovingly. 'I reckon that was the best meal we've ever had on *Earthrace*.'

I lie back looking at the stars. Lots are visible in the southern hemisphere and they're especially bright when out in the light-free wilderness like this. I start picking at a crayfish feeler, sucking out a long sliver of white and pink flesh. 'You know we are truly privileged to experience this,' I say to the lads. 'We live in the best country on earth. We've had amazing support from strangers all up and down the country . . . and we've visited the most stunning and remote parts of New Zealand.'

'Yeah and we've pigged out on some amazing seafood,' adds Ryan, holding up his plate and licking off the paua sauce.

We sit there for another hour soaking up an amazing evening, then set off for the long voyage north.

There's a noticeable difference between the east and west coasts of New Zealand. East coast beaches are pretty, with white sands, tame seas and generally easy harbour entrances. The west coast beaches are just the opposite, getting pummelled almost year round with big gnarly seas, and the entrances are littered with the wrecks of ships that have come to grief on the dangerous bars and reefs.

I look out the port window of *Earthrace* at Gannet Rock, just a few nautical miles away from us. I've dived and fished there with my brothers many times, and being here again is like coming home. Already I can detect the stench of seals and gannets, their guano covering the rocks. But it's almost appealing as I recognise the smell and associate it with home. I look down at the GPS, just 10 miles to go to Raglan, the last stop on our New Zealand tour. I pick up the VHF microphone and call the local Coastguard, who are coming out to guide us in over the notorious bar.

Sharyn and my two girls are waiting on the Golden Bay Wharf as we come in and dock. There's been a great team of volunteers organising things here, and already there's a solid group of people waiting to board *Earthrace*. 'Any sign of the kaumatua?' I ask John, as we're finalising the boarding plank.

'Yeah, he's just getting himself ready over there,' John says, pointing at an elderly man by the coffee cart. Hemi Rau of Tainui has been gracious enough to provide us with an elder to bless the boat, something we had missed in the mad dash of launching *Earthrace*. It feels like unfinished business, and I'm especially glad to have it done here on my home turf in Raglan. I wander over and introduce myself.

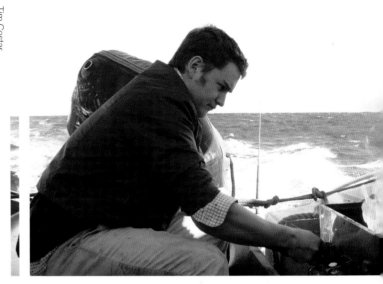

Tim Costar

Torsten getting the biodiesel cooker started. We got rid of it in the end. It was just too much hassle, and got dangerous in rough seas.

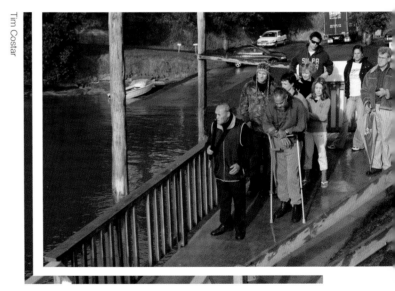

Tim Costar

Tainui kaumatua blessing *Earthrace* in Raglan. With me is Sharyn, Noel and Beverly Hunt (Sharyn's parents), my two girls Danielle and Alycia, plus crew Buddha and Ayla in the back. This was our last promotion in New Zealand before crossing the Pacific.

Five minutes later and he starts the blessing. It's an eerie mystical chant, as we gather behind him and start the slow walk down to *Earthrace*. It's like a prayer where you don't know the words, although you're still filled with a sense of spirit. He comes to the plank and ably walks over, despite the walking stick, and continues with the blessing. He reaches the cockpit and finishes, his final action being to strike the structure several times with his clenched fist.

The whole crew gather around and there's a real sense of unity among us. The blessing is like the final part of making *Earthrace* a genuine representative of New Zealand, and she can now leave our shores. Ryan has filmed the blessing and he's got a big grin on his face. 'Awesome bro.'

'Yeah. Feels like *Earthrace* is complete, eh?' We shake hands then wander back across the plank, John waiting patiently there with the first group of public ready to board.

## 'Yeah, no worries Pete, but if there's eight-metre waves, there's no way we'll be crossing the bar with ya'

The local Coastguard crew are waiting on the dock for a chat. 'There's a big storm brewing offshore Pete. If you're still leaving Monday, you'll likely have six- to eight-metre waves to battle. It might be better to wait a few days until she passes.'

I think about this for a minute. We've only had one decent storm, hardly enough to really test *Earthrace* in big seas, so I'd probably prefer to just head out and have it as part of the sea trials. It's better to find out any flaws in *Earthrace* here, rather than wait until we're in a storm half way across the Pacific.

'If we can get over the bar OK we'll just head out Monday as planned. You guys still OK to guide us out?'

'Yeah, no worries Pete, but if there's eight-metre waves, there's no way we'll be crossing the bar with ya.'

Monday arrives, and the voyage north turns into a nightmare, as we battle huge waves, several up to 12 metres in height, so we eventually seek shelter at Cornwallis in the Manukau Harbour. We wait a couple of days for

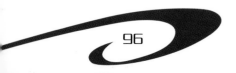

the waves to subside, before heading up to Cape Reinga and back down the east coast to Auckland.

I just arrive home when there's a call from Tourism New Zealand. They're threatening court action unless we remove the New Zealand map from the percentage symbol in our slogan '100% Pure Biodiesel'. You'd think they'd have better things to spend their time on than hassling us, I think after I've hung up. We've had no help from any government department whatsoever, and now one of them is threatening court action. They should be sponsoring us, not making our life difficult.

In terms of the public, though, our New Zealand tour has been a great success. We've had about 30,000 Kiwis walk aboard *Earthrace*, plus many, many more who have seen the boat on TV or in the newspapers. Most people around New Zealand now know the word biodiesel at least. And in terms of funds, when *Earthrace* was launched, we had about 200 grand in short-term debt, and this has now been reduced to only 50 grand. Thankfully, we relied on the public for this, and not a government department.

The big day to leave New Zealand finally arrives. We've stowed the life raft and the whole team is now busy loading the last of our supplies. The dock is full of family and friends waiting to see us off. Sharyn comes down and I hug her. I'm going to miss her and my two girls. I look over at Danielle and Alycia who are busy hassling Ryan about being a vegetarian. 'I'm going to call you Celery,' Alycia says to him cheekily. A tear rolls down my cheek. I feel like I'm deserting this wonderful family I've been blessed with. Sharyn suddenly bursts into tears. 'I love you and I'm going to miss you dreadfully,' she says between sobs.

'I love you too.' I hang onto her, not really wanting to leave but knowing I have to. I kiss her again then wander along the dock to board *Earthrace*. My throat aches and I start to cry as I clamber across the plank. I've travelled away from home many times, but this time it feels like it's for good. We give a final wave to everyone on shore, before we ease out of the dock, and on our way to Western Samoa.

There's a deep sense of loss at leaving my family behind. There's also a slight sense of trepidation, heading into the unknown. *Earthrace* has been right around New Zealand, but never more than about 30 miles offshore. Now we're on our way across the largest ocean on earth.

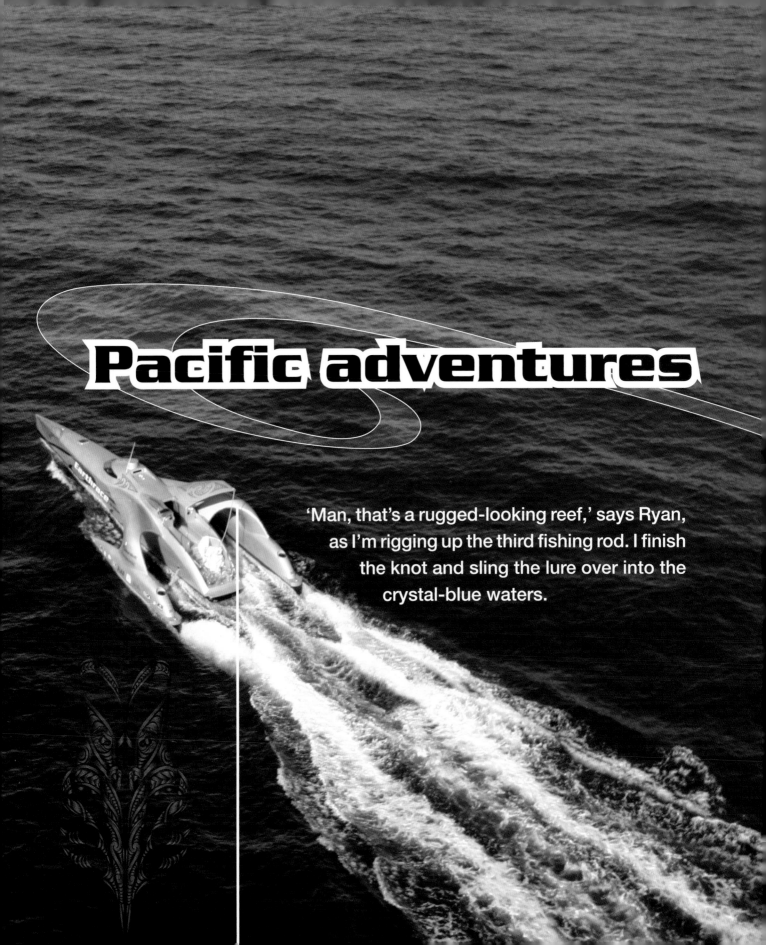

# Pacific adventures

'Man, that's a rugged-looking reef,' says Ryan, as I'm rigging up the third fishing rod. I finish the knot and sling the lure over into the crystal-blue waters.

'Yeah and probably full of fish, I reckon.' We're trolling at eight knots around South Minerva Reef, an amazing structure some 300 miles south of Western Samoa. I'm holding the rod feeding out line when there's a sudden explosion of water around the lure, and the line is ripped from my hand and starts disappearing from the reel. The fish has run about 50 metres before I engage the reel, the rod bends over taking the load, and then the line again peels off. A few seconds later and the fish is gone. I reel in the line to find it has chewed right through the leader. A new lure is put on and slung over the side.

Five minutes later and a huge marlin streaks through the water towards us, its streamlined fin slicing through the water. It nears the lures then suddenly veers off and disappears, before reappearing behind the lures. It makes a second run, this time nailing the green lure. The 24 kilo set suddenly bends over as the giant fish takes off, and the reel screams in protest.

'It's like trying to stop a horse,' I yell at Ryan, as I increase the drag until the braid is near breaking point.

The fish peels off about 300 metres of line then stops. I gain about 30 metres back on the now hot reel and then, amazingly, the fish just runs again until the reel is fully spooled, the line pinging as it reaches the end. I put the rod back in the holder, disappointed. 'Unbelievable. That marlin just spooled a fully loaded 24 kilo set. We're down to two lines guys,' I say, feeding out one of our two remaining sets.

# It's like trying to stop a horse, as I increase the drag until the braid is near breaking point

Both lures are side by side, and only 20 metres behind *Earthrace*. We have to watch for only a short time before a giant wahoo shoots out of the water with a lure in its mouth. Line peels off for a few seconds before the toothy beast chews through the leader. A few minutes later and a big yellowfin tuna grabs our one remaining lure. Torsten starts working the rod, but after a fight of around 10 minutes the hook pulls. We reset the line and it is hit by another giant wahoo, this time taking the lure with it.

'That's the last lure,' Torsten says, looking in our sad and empty tackle box.

'We'll just make one,' I say, grabbing some silicone tape from the workshop. We reshape a circle hook then tie some red and white silicone around it. The last of our trace line is tied on and we sling it over the side. Sure enough it's trolled for only a few minutes before it's hit by another wahoo. This time, though, the leader appears to hold. Ryan takes the rod and skilfully plays the fish, eventually easing it near the transom step, where Torsten waits and brings it aboard.

'Get a load of that!' yells Ryan in excitement, as we all admire his catch. Wahoo are unique among fish in that both their upper and lower jaws are hinged. I kneel down and look at the double sets of razor-sharp teeth. 'No wonder we lost so many lures with these critters out there.'

We fillet the fish, setting aside some for sashimi, some for dinner tonight and the balance we'll have over the next two days.

We head around the west side of the reef for a dive. 'You be careful here Pete,' says Paul Debenham (a volunteer from Tauranga) as I drop into the beautiful warm water. 'This area is loaded with sharks.' I look down and amazingly I can see the bottom already, and yet we're still in 30 metres of water. I swim slowly into the reef then drop down and hug the bottom. Gorgeous coral litter the reef structures, and there's a myriad of brightly coloured fish swimming around me. A couple of white-tip reef sharks come over and start to follow. Getting deeper, I start to see larger fish. A huge groper emerges from its hole, coming within a few feet and looking at me, before ambling back to his lair. Then a school of fish resembling red snapper, some as big as 15 kilograms, cruise past.

Paul has said to me the fish life in Minerva is fantastic. Being down here, though, it's almost unbelievable. The sheer size and variety of fish and coral make this one of the world's greatest dive spots and yet, because of its remoteness, hardly a soul ever gets here. Finally, a couple of larger sharks start sniffing around me so I decide to call it a day. I look up and there is *Earthrace*, its four-blade propellers spinning as the guys keep her away from the shallows. I start the slow ascent, anxious to keep an eye on the ever-present sharks. 'That is the most amazing dive I've ever had,' I say to the guys as I clamber onto the transom step.

We make our way to Western Samoa where we restock *Earthrace* with food, fuel and water. We then head back out to sea, en route to Hawaii. 'Man it's getting hot,' complains Ryan. He's taken his shirt off and is sweating profusely. He looks like a praying mantis, with his long limbs draped all over the navigator's chair. I look back at the helm temperature gauge and see it's 35 degrees.

'How about a swim?' I suggest.

'Better still, how about a wakeboard?' Ryan says. He suddenly perks up and scampers forward to grab the wakeboard Rebel Sport had given us a few months earlier.

I jump in the water and grab the ski rope, then tuck my legs up to keep the board facing *Earthrace*. Ryan talks on the radio to Ove, a Swedish guy crewing for us at the moment, who is driving. There's the roar as 1080 horsepower kicks into gear and the rope goes tight. Within a second or two I'm standing up as the wakeboard skims over the surface. I veer left and right a few times, before canning off over the wake, with the lads on the stern all laughing.

*Earthrace* seems like a long way off by the time she finally stops. I feel very vulnerable just sitting here in five-mile-deep water and with nothing around. Strange, really, because I'm safer here than close to reefs or islands, where there are more likely to be big sharks lurking. *Earthrace* backs up and I have another go, this time staying on a bit longer, before falling off trying to jump the wake.

Paul has just finished his turn when Ove comes running out to the cockpit. 'The water bladder has burst,' he says in a thick Swedish accent. We go inside and sure enough the fresh water bladder under the helm floor has split, the water now sloshing around in the confined compartment. I scoop up a cupful and swirl it around in my mouth. There's a horrible chemical taste about it, and I end up spitting it out. 'That water for sure is stuffed,' I say to the guys, who now all look very worried. 'With the two spare

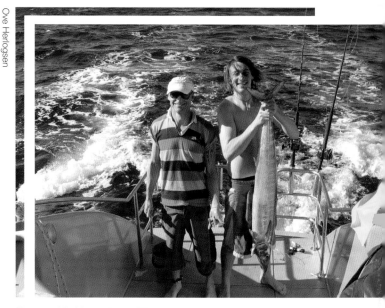

Ryan with his wahoo. This was caught at Minerva Reef, some 300 nautical miles south of Western Samoa. The most amazing reef I've ever seen, and absolutely teeming with fish.

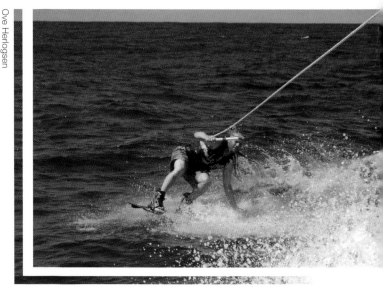

Paul Debenham wakeboarding in the middle of the Pacific. It is very unnerving when you fall off in five-mile deep water waiting to be picked back up.

containers, we've got enough for a couple of days only, and yet we're three days from Hawaii.' Ryan heads over to the GPS system and starts looking at islands.

'Hey, there's an atoll directly in our path, although I can't tell if it is inhabited or not.' I look down at the GPS. Palmyra Atoll. I've never heard of it before. It has a couple of very straight shorelines, which are probably man-made. So it's likely there are people and water there.

We start debating what it'll be like. 'I think I've heard of it before,' says Paul. 'It's an abandoned military base.' Torsten reckons it's completely

# Once we get to within 30 miles away I call on the VHF hoping to reach someone

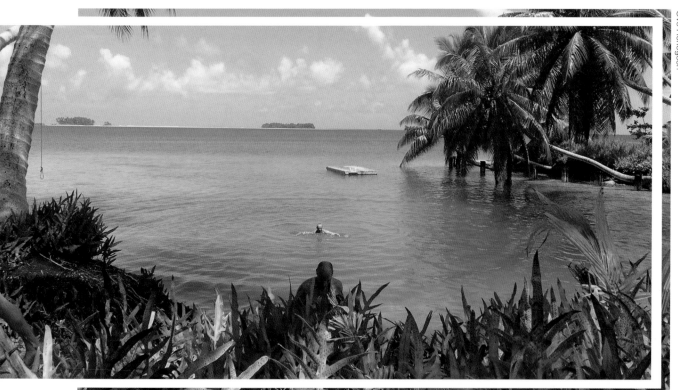

Ove Herlogsen

Palmyra Atoll, a day or two south of Hawaii. We had a quick swim in this watering hole before heading back to sea. One of the best-kept secrets in the Pacific.

barren with no water, while Ryan thinks it'll just have a few islanders living there. The speculation continues about what the island will be like, and what we'll do if there isn't any water there.

It's a precarious position to be in. One minute we're rolling along with 240 litres of water, and the next we're down to 40. Maybe the bladders are not such a good idea after all. That one broke in pretty benign conditions. I look down at the mysterious Palmyra Atoll on the GPS again. Another 24 hours and we should be there.

Once we get to within 30 miles away I call on the VHF hoping to reach someone.

'Palmyra Atoll, Palmyra Atoll, this is *Earthrace*, *Earthrace*, do you copy? Over.' Everyone crowds around, anxious to know if there are people living on the island.

There's a long delay before a muffled American voice comes back, '*Earthrace*, this is Palmyra Atoll, go ahead, over.'

'We are a vessel en route to Hawaii, our water bladder has burst, we have only one day's supply left, and we would like to come in and land on Palmyra Atoll to get fresh water please, over.'

'Negative Captain, you do not have permission to land on Palmyra Atoll. This is a US wildlife sanctuary and it is illegal for you to land here. Please make other arrangements. Over.'

I call him back and explain we really need the water, but he is adamant we cannot land. We all sit there amazed that they wouldn't let us in.

Going back to the charts, there are a couple of islands 150 nautical miles east of our location that will definitely have water, but it is a long way off our course to Hawaii.

'What about we just sneak in and get what we need,' Ryan suggests.

'Yeah, in the *Earthrace* stealth boat; they'll never notice us,' says Torsten sarcastically.

'The only way we'd get in without being spotted is after dark, but I wouldn't want to do that just relying on charts. For us to land it'd need to be in daylight.'

'Maybe we go to the second uninhabited atoll, and if there's no water supply, we'll just grab coconuts,' Ryan suggests.

The VHF crackles back at us. 'This is Palmyra Atoll. You have permission to land. Please radio us when you reach the harbour and we will escort you in.' There's high fives all around as we change course back to the harbour.

Palmyra here we come. Although why they suddenly changed their minds remains a mystery.

The atoll typifies what I'd imagined a tropical paradise to look like. Beautiful blue water, a sheltered lagoon, coconut trees hanging out over the water and lush tropical forest away from the water's edge. 'This is paradise,' Ove says. He's on the bow checking for reefs, as we idle into the lagoon.

We make it to shore, and are escorted into the cafeteria, where a group of about 20 people are having lunch. A Kiwi bloke approaches us and explains that he'd taken his son aboard *Earthrace* in Wellington, and he's got one of our signed posters hanging on his wall. When he heard it was *Earthrace* wanting to come in here, he hassled the park ranger who eventually agreed to give us permission. It turns out there are seven researchers here from New Zealand, all keen to meet us. It's a small world when you're a Kiwi.

After lunch we have a swim in their watering hole and then load up with water and some fresh bread. A bikini-clad girl comes up as we're filling the last of the containers. She's got a deep tan that comes from spending most of the day scantily clad, and her legs and arms are lean and muscular.

'Um. A few of us were wondering if we could, you know, have a look in your boat?'

I look over at Ryan who raises his eyebrows and smiles.

'Yeah, no worries,' I say. 'Ryan and Torsten here will give you all a personal, guided tour.' They jump into the small tender and shuttle out to *Earthrace*. Fifteen minutes later and they're still not back. I look over and Ryan is busy selling them T-shirts on the back deck. Nice one.

We're all buzzing as we leave the atoll.

'What a wicked place that was,' says Ryan, as he's munching on a slice of fresh bread and hummus.

The island disappears behind us, as we set a course for Maui in Hawaii. 'Can you believe Palmyra has only 21 people, and I managed to sell 19 T-shirts,' says Ryan, digging a fistful of US and Kiwi money out of his pocket.

# North America
## – west coast

It's a stunning day that greets us in Vancouver. *Earthrace* is docked in a great little spot on Granville Island, although I'm still anxious about how things will go. West Coast Reduction is sponsoring us, and they've organised all the media, but we have no idea what networks are coming down or what we can expect. All we know is we must have *Earthrace* and ourselves on the dock at 1pm. I pull my cell phone out: almost one o'clock already.

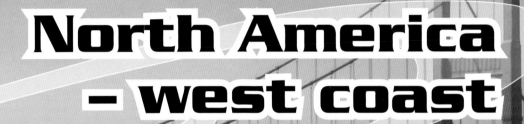

100% PURE BIODIESEL *Earthrace*

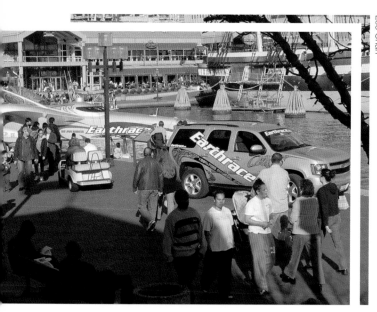

Leo Chan

An open day in Baltimore. Check out the Earthrace car, compliments of David and Marta Perez.

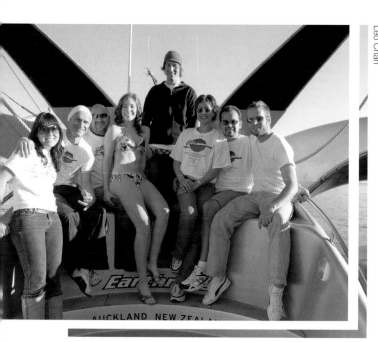

Leo Chan

Posing with the crew in Baltimore. Left to right: Devann, myself, John, a local swimsuit model, Ryan, Marta Perez, David Perez, Mike Scheeman.

A local comes over, looking interested. 'You involved with this, ay?' he asks, pointing at *Earthrace*. He's got that Canadian 'ay' thing going on at the end of his sentences.

'Yep. What would you like to know?'

'Well, for a start, what's this biodiesel stuff all about, ay?'

I launch into my usual spiel I've given a hundred times back in New Zealand. 'It's a renewable fuel made from vegetable oils or animal fats, and it can run in most modern diesel engines. The fuel is renewable and has reduced emissions in almost all categories compared with petro-diesel. It saves your foreign exchange reserves because the fuel is purchased locally, rather than sending funds off to the Middle East.'

'There are regional employment advantages, because you tend to have small factories scattered around the country, rather than a single refinery. It is also a labour-intensive rather than capital-intensive industry. This results in increased employment . . . and the fuel is nearly carbon neutral.' The guy raises his hand to stop me.

'Carbon neutral? How can that be? Surely if you burn the fuel, you release carbon dioxide?'

I explain that the carbon dioxide emitted when the fuel is burned is balanced by the carbon dioxide that is trapped by plants the fuel is made from. He looks at me confused. In fact it is not entirely carbon neutral, because you require energy to process the fuel, but in terms of greenhouse gas emissions, biodiesel is way better than petro-diesel.

A film crew arrives and are setting up down by *Earthrace*, so I excuse myself and head down.

'Who are you guys with?' I ask, looking at their old Beta cameras. The local has followed me down and is watching on.

'We're with the Canadian Broadcasting Corporation,' one of them says. We complete the interview, which is to be broadcast nationally in Canada. Then a local Vancouver crew arrives, and after this a crew from Shaw TV, followed by newspaper and radio journalists. It's late afternoon before we finish with the last photographer.

With such a good media turnout and great location, Vancouver is a huge success for us, as is Seattle a few days later. From there we head down to Portland in Oregon, a city some 90 miles inland from the coast. We enter the harbour and start our slow voyage up the Columbia River, passing under the Astoria Bridge just on dusk. 'What's he up to do ya reckon?' I say to Ryan, pointing at a small stationary boat right on the edge of the shipping lane.

# Torsten grabs a knife, jumps into the water and starts cutting us free

'Maybe a fisherman or a water taxi.'

Ryan spots a couple of small buoys in the water pointing back towards the boat, and we suddenly realise he's strung a net right across the shipping lane, and directly in our path. I take *Earthrace* out of gear but it's too late, as we drift over the top of his net, our propellers and rudders all getting tangled up.

'There's a ship right up our backside,' yells Torsten, pointing to a bulk carrier looming up behind us.

Torsten grabs a knife, jumps into the water and starts cutting us free, while I radio the ship behind us alerting them that we're disabled. They don't respond, so I just assume they haven't heard, and head out the back to help Torsten.

By now the small fishing boat is alongside us. 'You can't sling a bloody net right across the shipping lane,' I yell at him. He's trying to recover sections of net as Torsten hacks them to bits. He shrugs his shoulders but doesn't say anything. I glance back at the bulk carrier, by now just 400 metres behind us. 'Only the starboard rudder to go,' Torsten yells. I'm about to tie a line to the small fishing boat to tow us out of the boat's path, when Torsten yells, 'All clear Pete,' as he throws the last bit of net at the fisherman and jumps onto our transom step. *Earthrace* is thrown into gear and we accelerate out of harm's way, watching the huge bulk carrier as it goes by. 'Where'd he go?' says Ryan, as we try to locate the fisherman. 'Looks like he's done a runner.'

The voyage up the Columbia River is slow, tedious and stressful, as we weave our way around boats of all shapes and sizes working through the night. Our shifts are two hours on and two hours off, with two people on the helm at each time. Ryan and I have just taken over at 3am and the river looks clear when a bunch of white lights start appearing on the corner ahead of us. 'Here they are,' says Ryan, pointing at a big blob on the radar moving our way.

I pick up the binoculars, and spot three vertical lights on the masthead. 'Looks like a vessel under tow.' We head towards the starboard side of the lane, but the towing vessel is gradually drifting into our path. I call them on the radio but there's no response.

## We're suddenly blinded from a spotlight on a small boat, then the radio squawks

'Get the others up Ryan. This is starting to get tricky.' By now the blob on the radar has morphed into four different blobs moving about, and it's clear they're going to take up the entire lane and then some. We slow down and angle dangerously close to the starboard bank, as the tow vessel continues its relentless course towards us.

We're suddenly blinded from a spotlight on a small boat, then the radio squawks. '*Earthrace, Earthrace*, can you please turn around and pass us on the port side? Over.' I look at the narrow area to work with. They're only 30 seconds from us, nowhere near enough time to turn around in.

'Negative sir. We are unable to turn around. Please move as far to starboard as you can to pass us on your port side. Over.'

There's no reply, and the group of boats just continue towards us, as we drive closer to the bank. We're in only a metre or so of water by now. Ryan suddenly spots something ahead and yells to stop, but it's too late and there's the sickening sound of breaking carbon as our main bow hits something solid.

'Back it up Pete!' Ryan yells, but I'm reluctant to go back too far or we'll be hit by the tow vessel. So we stay there like sitting ducks.

A tugboat passes us, blinding us again with a spotlight. It's hard to tell exactly what they're towing. Maybe a house on a giant barge. The barge passes, coming within about four metres of us, and then there's another barge being towed by the first, this one perilously close to us. 'It's going to be real close,' yells Ryan as it drifts in. They've got a smaller boat on its stern trying to pull it away from us but with little effect. It drifts by, missing our port sponson by centimetres. 'Man, that was scary,' says Ryan with obvious relief as he comes back into the helm. 'Can you believe they were actually towing two barges behind that tugboat?'

We're a tired crew that finally pull into Portland around lunchtime, and survey the big chunk of carbon taken out of our bow. The good thing is we were only doing a couple of knots, so the damage is mostly cosmetic. Our local volunteer Brian Van Buskirk is there to meet us, and he's organised several events over our four-day stop. One of these is an auction where they sell off various items of donated goods, as well as a sunset cruise up the Willamette River on *Earthrace*. It's late on Saturday evening when we set off on the cruise, with around 15 local people who have paid to join our mostly Kiwi crew. They sit on the roof of *Earthrace*, drinking and smoking as we make our way upstream.

'You've got to be pretty wealthy to own a home up here,' Brian says, as we pass a group of huge riverfront properties with large stately houses nestled among manicured lawns, swimming pools and tennis courts.

'Oh check out that fat-cat house,' I say, pointing to an enormous mansion about double the size of the rest. There are a couple of bouncy castles with kids running around them, and some adults sitting by a pool sipping drinks. Off the end of the property is a small dock.

'Shall we see if we can go ashore?' I say to Brian.

'What do you mean?'

'Well, we'll dock behind their boat and have a play on their bouncy castles and stuff. It'll be a laugh.'

'They'll never let you in. They'll probably shoot you for illegally entering their property.'

'Nah mate. This is *Earthrace*.'

Torsten grabs the wheel and I get up on the horn of *Earthrace* and jump in, swimming over to their dock.

A couple of adults come running down, a short guy by the name of Roger glaring at me as I clamber up.

'I was wondering if I pull my boat in to your dock, your kids can play on it for a while, and we'll go and play on your bouncy castles?' Roger's eyes open wide and he stares at me for a second.

'Where are you from?'

'I'm from New Zealand, and our boat is attempting a round the world speed record next year . . . and we fuel the boat on biodiesel.'

'Oh my God! That is so cool,' says the middle-aged lady hanging off his arm. 'Yeah, what the hell,' he replies, offering me his hand. 'Come ashore and join the party.'

*Earthrace* is docked and our guests and crew all disgorge into the huge compound. There's free wine and beer being served, bouncy castles to jump on, and a heated 20-metre pool to hang out in. The kids disappear into *Earthrace* for half an hour while we meet the parents, who are clearly all very wealthy. The Kiwi crew then start a bombing competition, and before long we're up on the second storey of the house jumping into the enormous pool, parents busy

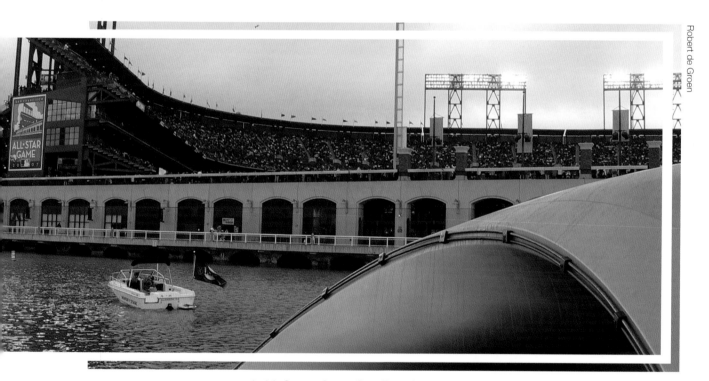

Robert de Groen

In McCovey Cove, San Francisco, with the ball park in the background. Big hits can end up in the water around you. Shots of us were beamed nationwide during this ball game.

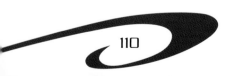

trying to keep their kids from following our unwanted example.

It turns into a crazy wild night, and it's 3am before we gather all our guests back onto *Earthrace* and undock. Our hosts had bought over 600 bucks' worth of T-shirts and posters, then handed over a thousand dollars and said to keep the change. They welcomed us into their home and their circle of friends and were impeccably nice to us, despite our running amok.

Portland is a great little promotion, but San Francisco by contrast is disappointing. Local media for some reason have not been very interested. We've had the amazing situation of a *New York Times* reporter coming down to write a story, and yet the local *San Francisco Chronicle* said they were too busy. It's also hard for the public to find us, as we're tucked behind fences, barriers and security, away from the public gaze. Many US docks are becoming like fortresses as they erect fences and barriers in the wake of 9/11.

The main highlight in San Francisco is taking *Earthrace* into McCovey Cove, which is beside the Giants' Baseball Park. A game is in progress and the cameras fix on us a number of times and John Miller, the commentator, starts talking about *Earthrace* on his nationwide broadcast. Traffic on our website goes ballistic, until the server finally crashes from overload.

We spend the first couple of nights sleeping on the floor of the Pier 39 offices, until John finally scores a couple of sponsored rooms at a nearby hotel. I've now got Ryan and Torsten in my room, thankfully far away from John, who snores, scratches and moans incessantly at night. It's 3am and I look out the window to see *Earthrace* coming off its ropes, so I wake Ryan and ask him to go and sort it out. He runs off down the hall in his underwear. I jump back into bed, but in the back of my mind I'm uneasy about something, although I'm not quite sure what.

Ryan has run half way to the boat when a patrol car pulls alongside him. The officer shines his torch at Ryan, no doubt curious why he'd be running along in his undies at three in the morning. 'What are you up to then?'

'Oh, our boat is tied up at Pier 39 but it's come off its ropes, so I'm just going to sort it out.' The officer looks at Ryan for a long time then drives off, shaking his head. By now Ryan is just starting to wake up, but cannot quite figure it out. He arrives to find *Earthrace* sitting nicely alongside the dock and still tied off. He looks back towards our hotel, over a mile away, and cannot even see it. How the hell did Pete see the boat from there he wonders? He decides to just sleep on *Earthrace* rather than run all the way back to the hotel.

The following morning Torsten sheds some light. Apparently I was sleepwalking, and I'd started cursing and swearing about *Earthrace* coming loose, but I was staring at the blank wall in our room. Ryan, also a sleepwalker, had stood there beside me looking at the wall, and believing that, yes, *Earthrace* was indeed coming loose. And with that he'd disappeared out of the room in his underwear to sort the problem.

From San Francisco we start a magical part of the tour through the rest of California, visiting Monterey, Morro Bay, Santa Cruz, Santa Barbara, Ventura, Newport, Redondo Beach, San Diego, Oceanside, Long Beach and finishing in Marina Del Ray, the last stop on our west coast tour. We've just finished filming with a local crew when John comes running over very excited.

'You know that company Better Biodiesel I've been talking to?'

'Mmm. Not really.'

'Well, they're a small start-up company in Utah that has developed a new process for making biodiesel.' It seems every company you meet in the biodiesel industry is claiming a new process that is better than all the rest. 'Well, they've agreed to sponsor us all the biodiesel fuel for the race. They'll ship it for us, and they're chipping in ten grand US a month for the next year.' John understandably has a big grin on his face, and there are high fives all round. I don't really care if they have a new process or not. If they're doing all that for us they're OK by me.

There's a renewed sense of optimism among us as *Earthrace* leaves Los Angeles and heads down to Panama. To have all our fuel sorted will make funding the race much easier. Plus the cash each month will be fantastic.

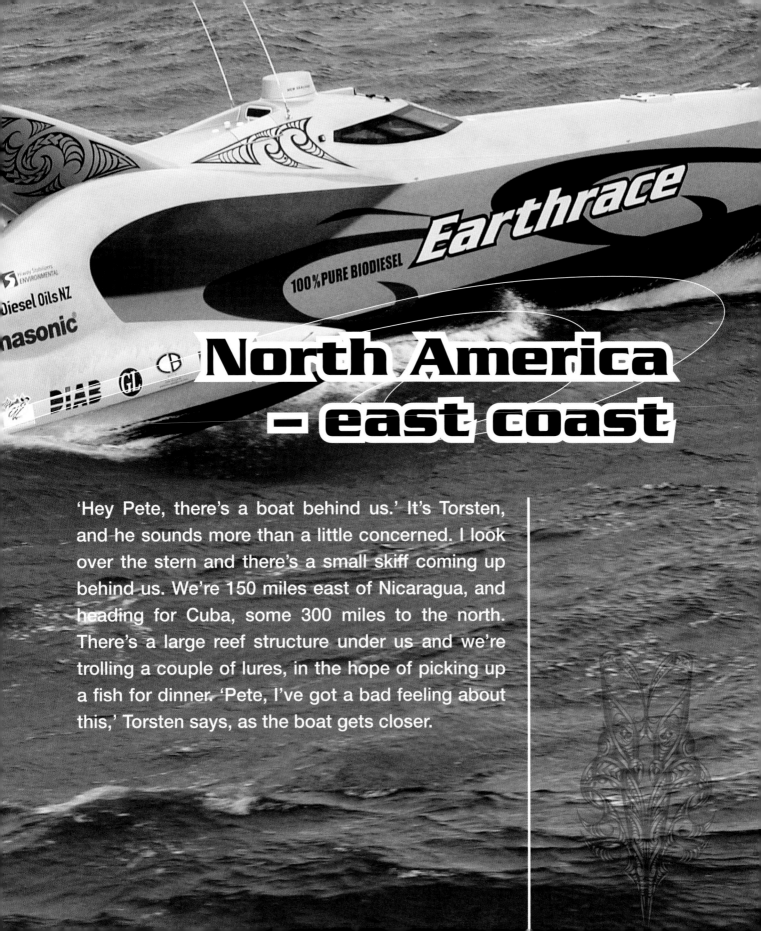

# North America – east coast

'Hey Pete, there's a boat behind us.' It's Torsten, and he sounds more than a little concerned. I look over the stern and there's a small skiff coming up behind us. We're 150 miles east of Nicaragua, and heading for Cuba, some 300 miles to the north. There's a large reef structure under us and we're trolling a couple of lures, in the hope of picking up a fish for dinner. 'Pete, I've got a bad feeling about this,' Torsten says, as the boat gets closer.

He's always needlessly worrying about things, I think to myself, but I pick up the binoculars and take a look anyway. Just a little fishing boat I reckon, although there are a lot of guys in it. Thirty seconds later, though, and I can just make out what look like a couple of guns.

'Let's clear the lines Torst. Maybe you're right.' Ryan pushes both throttles forward while Torsten and I pull in the two lures, now skipping along on the surface as we accelerate over 25 knots. The skiff by now is practically right on top of us, smoke billowing out of its little outboard engine. We scarper back inside and I grab the VHF.

'This is *Earthrace, Earthrace*. The small skiff on our starboard side, what are your intentions? Over.'

A scratchy voice comes back in Spanish but none of us can understand what he's saying.

'Englese perfavore,' I reply, which translates as 'English please', about my sum total of Spanish.

# 'They're bloody pirates, I told ya we should've left when we had the chance'

There's a long silence. I can see the boat now about 50 metres from our starboard window. There are five guys aboard, four of them carrying what look like M16 assault rifles.

'They've got guns,' I say to the crew, who are all anxiously huddled in the helm.

'They're bloody pirates,' replies Torsten. 'I told ya we should've left when we had the chance.'

One of the pirates is lying on the bow with his rifle pointed directly at us. The VHF crackles but it's such a dodgy signal we can hardly make out what they're saying.

'I think they're saying they're the Colombian navy,' Ryan says.

'Repeat perfavore,' I reply.

'This Colombian navy. Stop now or we shoot.'

I look again at the small skiff. No markings at all and blowing smoke. It hardly looks like a navy vessel. No uniforms that I can make out.

'Negative sir, we will not stop for you. Your boat has no markings and we do not believe you are navy, over.'

I've just finished my sentence when there's an audible thud, as a bullet hits *Earthrace*. We all look at each other in horror.

'Get behind the spars!' I yell at the crew, who all scamper behind the big carbon structures in the galley. They're 66 layers thick and effectively bulletproof.

By now my mind is racing from the terrifying situation we're suddenly in. If they're pirates, they'll either be robbing us or taking hostages. Either way it's bad news. We can certainly outrun them, and already they're starting to fall behind, although if they all opened fire our fuel tanks would be poked full of holes. We'd still have enough to make it to shore somewhere, though. I'd rather be in port with no fuel than have my crew taken hostage by these dudes.

I look down at the GPS. There is a shallow reef coming up, so I set the autopilot to turn to starboard avoiding it. Unfortunately, it also brings us back closer to the pirates who are off to that side. I look over at the skiff and see a white flash from the muzzle; a split second later the second bullet rips into our hull. A beautiful sunny day has turned into an absolute nightmare.

The VHF crackles. 'Captain, Captain. How many crew?'

Which surprises me. Firstly, he called me 'Captain', which is more a military or coastguard response. And, secondly, he wants to know how many crew, again typical of the military who have set procedures they follow for boarding a vessel, one of which is accounting for all the crew. I'm starting to think maybe they are military after all. That boat, though, sure doesn't look like navy.

I pick up the radio. 'Can you tell me what vessel you are over from?' If it is a navy vessel, he'll have a frigate or patrol boat somewhere around here that he's come from. His response comes back immediately, and it's difficult to tell exactly what he says. Perhaps the *Quintos*. I'm not really sure, but he answered straight away, which suggests he's not making it up at least.

I look back at the crew, all cowering behind the spars. Either I jump back there with them now and we ride out the imminent hailstorm of bullets, or we stop now and hope they really are navy. Ryan amazingly has been filming right through this, and he's pointing the camera at Torsten who looks petrified. 'I'm going to stop guys. I don't know if they are navy or not, but I think we should stop.'

I pull the throttles back to neutral, while the skiff circles us then approaches the stern. As they come in, I can see several of them looking down their rifle sights at us. Please be navy, please be navy, I keep saying to myself. 'No film, no film,' the head guys yells at Ryan, who diligently sits his camera down on the step, but leaves it rolling. They're a motley-looking bunch. The head guy has a pistol at his side and his hand is on the holster, while all the others are carrying M16 assault rifles. A few of them are wearing what could be considered a uniform. They're also all wearing the same caps. The head guy steps aboard and glares at me menacingly. 'I Lieutenant Chavez of Colombia navy. Where your papers?' Torsten scurries forward to get our clearance papers from Panama, as well as our New Zealand registration certificate.

Chavez stands there with his hands on his hips, looking us over. 'Bring me your guns and drugs,' he demands. I explain that we don't have any guns or drugs aboard, but he's unconvinced. He barks some orders at one of his men, who scurries forward and starts searching.

## 'Look at your boat, Lieutenant, it sure doesn't look like a navy boat to me'

'And why you not stop when ordered?' he asks me.

'Look at your boat, Lieutenant, it sure doesn't look like a navy boat to me,' and I point at his little skiff spluttering away behind us.

A wry smile crosses his face and he looks up at me. 'In Colombia, this a *good* navy vessel,' and he chuckles at his joke.

It turns out they are from a patrol boat anchored on the other side of the reef. The US Drug Enforcement Agency funds them to patrol these waters, picking up traffickers taking drugs from Colombia and Brazil up to Florida, and the route we're on is apparently State Highway One for drug smuggling.

Chavez and his crew continue their search and find nothing, eventually leaving us, but taking with them a couple of signed posters and a DVD. As their little skiff heads off, we sit there looking at each other, just thankful to be alive and free. One minute we were cruising along enjoying the sun and thinking about fresh sashimi, the next we're looking down the barrels of a bunch of assault rifles. 'How about a swim?' says Ryan, and he runs up the horn and jumps into the water, shrieking, 'It's good to be alive!' on the way down. We have a quick swim, but are keen to get away before the Colombians change their minds. No fish for dinner but, man, it is good to be alive.

We pass the west coast of Cuba without incident then head up to the Fort Lauderdale Boat Show. From there the tour kicks into gear. We visit Boston, Newport, New York, Philadelphia, Indian River Marina, Baltimore, Hilton Head, Wilmington, Savannah, Key West, Jacksonville, St Petersburg, Tampa, Houston, New Orleans, Mobile, Pensacola and Destin. We then head to Charleston in South Carolina, where Cummins Mercruiser is based, and we pull *Earthrace* from the water to do some final preparations before the race.

The refit period is a total of three weeks, making it by far the longest time we've been in one city since *Earthrace* was launched. 'It's like having a home again, eh?' says John as we sit down at the table to a plate of muesli. I scan the room and it looks like a scene from *Animal House*. Unwashed dishes litter the bench and tables, and clothing, blankets and suitcases cover the floor. Bodies are huddled inside sleeping bags and blankets. By the door is a

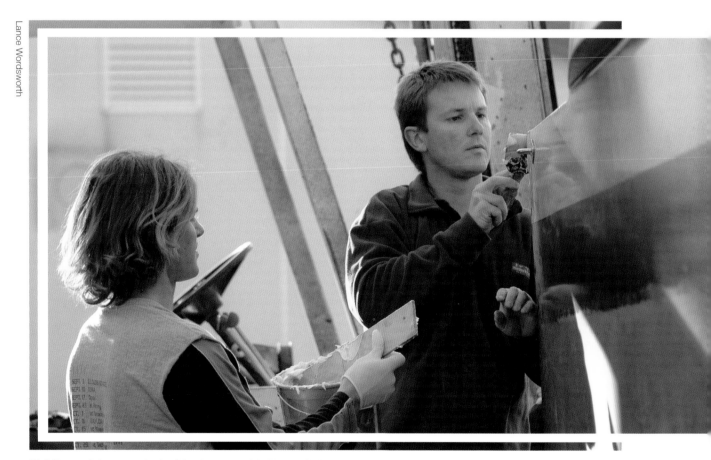

Lance Wordsworth

Phil Ross doing repairs in Charleston, with Ryan Kiefer assisting.

mountain of beer and wine bottles, but more worryingly, there's the stench of something rotten. John screws his nose up. 'Phew, something sure travels in here.'

'We've got another warning,' says Devann, who's been handling our media and PR for the last four months. 'What for this time?' I ask. It'll be our fifth warning since we got here three weeks ago.

'Loud parties,' and she hands me an official warning letter from the body corporate that looks after the units. 'Were we loud last night? I can't really remember.' Judging by my hangover maybe we did get a bit out of control.

'Loud?' laughs Devann. 'You damned Kiwis were playing rugby in the carpark at four this morning, and then you decided to have a skateboarding competition.' A bit of it starts to come back to me. We went to some Coyote Ugly bar in town and ended up drinking vodka and Red Bulls, and then came home pissed but full of energy.

Ryan stirs on the floor. He's lying in his sleeping bag with a plate of food by his pillow, and scraps that didn't quite make it to his mouth scattered around him. 'Oh what a wicked hangover,' he says, squinting between half open eyes. 'I'm not really sure I'm up to that game of rugby today.'

I'd forgotten about that. We were having the morning off today, playing some USA versus New Zealand games down at the park.

'Without wishing to sound like your mom,' says Devann, 'we need to clean this place up before we head off anywhere. Jeff McDermott has been overly generous in loaning us this house, but right now we're just trashing it.'

'Oh, you're so cute when you're angry,' John says to her lovingly, and wraps a big hairy arm around her neck.

'Um, Pete. Is this a good time to talk about money?' John asks, turning back to me and suddenly looking serious.

'As good as any.'

'Look, I just don't know where the race money is going to come from. With Better Biodiesel going under, I reckon we'll need at least a quarter million to run the race. And right now we only have about thirty grand.'

We found out a short time ago that Better Biodiesel's funding has dried up, and it seems likely they're going to go bust, which of course means they'll not be sponsoring us the fuel and cash they'd committed to.

'You know, I reckon we should concentrate on getting separate companies to sponsor the fuel for individual race legs. We've spent the last six months promoting biodiesel all over North America, so I'm sure some biodiesel companies here will be willing to sponsor us fuel. Maybe concentrate on Barbados, Panama, Acapulco and San Diego initially, because we'll need these first when we start the race. As for the money, I'm not sure where it'll come from, but I know we'll just piece it together like we always do.'

John looks unconvinced.

'What about we delay the race until later in the year, to give us time to get the extra funds?'

Ryan by now has spotted the plate of food beside him and is picking at it. 'If we don't leave by mid March, we'll lose the weather window and have to delay a whole year.'

'Well, maybe that's what we should do,' John says.

'Look, John. We've made commitments to sponsors and supporters that we'll run the race next month, and that's what we're going to do. The fuel and funding will come, but we need to work on it now, and we need to have faith that it will happen.'

'Yeah, John. Just have faith,' Ryan says mockingly.

John rolls his eyes, and goes back to his muesli.

We muster up the whole gang and amazingly there are 16 of us sleeping in a little three-bedroom unit that has been loaned to us. This refit has been a revelation in terms of volunteers. Allison and Scott travelled all the way from Panama to join us. Ryan Kiefer drove over a thousand miles from Nebraska. There's a group of composite experts from Philadelphia, plus a couple of lads from New York. Originally, I thought we'd run out of time here, but at the moment we're actually ahead of schedule in terms of work on *Earthrace*.

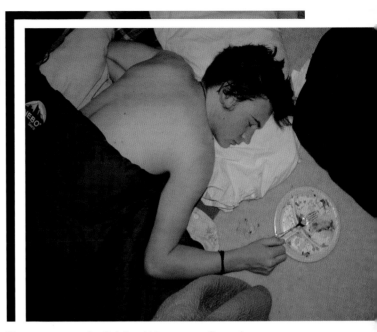

Ryan never quite finished his graze after a heavy night out.

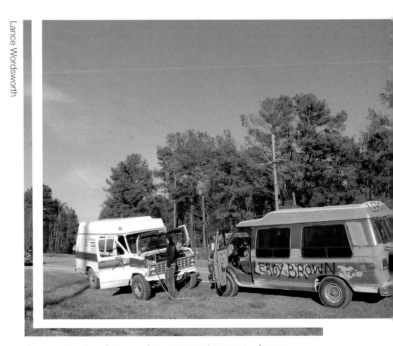

Jump-starting Leroy after we ran her out of gas in Charleston.

We clean the unit as best you can with 16 people living there, then squeeze into Leroy, a V8 Chevy van that was given to us by a volunteer in Miami a few months back. Most of us are still sporting hangovers, but with breakfast and a crisp sunny day we're all coming right. The prospect of a game of rugby starts to appeal, especially the chance to kick a few US butts. The Americans, though, are having nothing to do with rugby, so we borrow a soccer ball from a family nearby and have a go at that. The Kiwis clean up five–nil, then we set up for a game of bullrush. 'These Yanks are useless, eh?' says John, as we're marking out the area. 'I mean they could hardly kick a ball to save themselves.' Actually, it seems like we're either really good

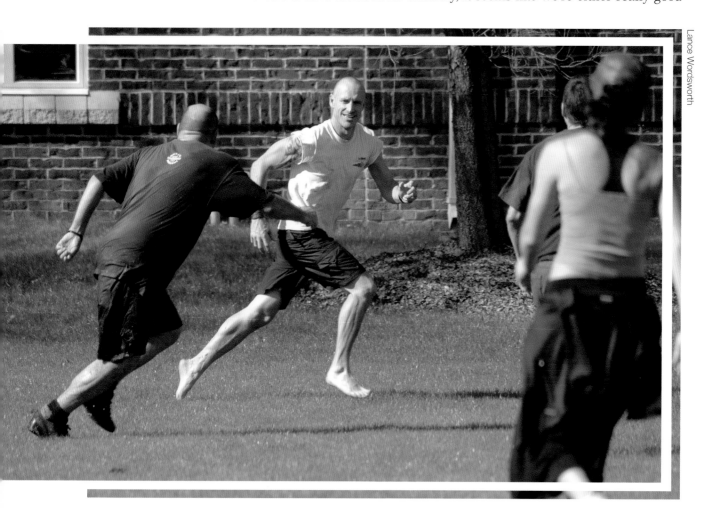

Lance Wordsworth

John lining up to tackle me in the game of bullrush. He can't quite run an 11-second 100 m dash any more. Devann and Anthony to the right.

or they're really useless. A couple of their guys clearly spend a lot of time in the gym, but it sure hasn't helped their soccer skills. Bullrush is more of the same. The Americans just get targeted early because they are so easy to tackle, and so easy to escape from if they are after you.

It's a tired crew that arrives at the boatyard a few hours later, various bruises starting to make themselves known. *Earthrace* is up on blocks, and she's an impressive beast out of the water. 'They're the weirdest looking props I've ever seen,' Scott yells at me, as he's unpacking the new carbon propellers that arrived the day before.

'Well, they might look weird but, according to Loomes, they'll give us at least another knot or two of speed.' The theory is the carbon blades flex under load; they're supposedly more efficient and less prone to vibrations. Scott kneels down and lifts up the starboard prop and slides it onto the shaft. 'Well, I don't know if they'll be faster, but they sure are light.'

I climb up into *Earthrace* and down into the engine room. The Cummins Mercruiser team have given the engines a full inspection, and changed out various bits and pieces. 'You going to be ready to go back in the water tomorrow?' I ask Anthony, who is busy sorting all the spare engine parts.

'Yeah, sweet as. Ready now, actually. A bit concerned about spare parts, though. We're still missing the turbocharger, pistons and head gaskets.'

'Just follow up with Cummins. I'm sure they'll sort them before we leave.'

I clamber down and wander around *Earthrace*. Amazingly, we'll have everything organised by the time the cranes arrive tomorrow to lift *Earthrace* back in the water. My talk with John earlier in the day sits uneasily in the back of my mind, however. Getting *Earthrace* to the start line in Barbados on 10 March will be easy from here. But having all the race fuel and funds ready in time is another matter.

The next day *Earthrace* is lowered back into the water, and from there we head down to the Miami Boat Show, and then across to Puerto Rico, a couple of days east of Miami. This stop turns out to be our most successful ever, with fantastic sponsors, great media support and an enormous number of people through the boat. We sign up a new sponsor called Ciclon, who are the leading energy drink supplier in the Caribbean and Central America. 'We'd like you to have our logo on the side of your boat,' their marketing manager said to me during negotiations, 'plus we'd like you to take one of our models with you on a leg of the race.'

'You mean, someone like her,' I reply, pointing to one of their young ladies who's been handing out Ciclon drinks. She's a curvaceous young Puerto Rican in an impossibly tight Lycra outfit with carefully selected cut-outs. John is busy having his photo taken with the stunning model.

'Yes. Someone like her.'

She can come for free, I'm thinking, and I glance over at Ryan who's got a big cheeky smile on his face. We finalise details, agreeing that, weather and safety concerns permitting, we'll take the model on the last leg of the race, from the Canary Islands to Barbados. In exchange, we get a much-

# 'You know, I still can't quite believe that this time tomorrow we'll actually be racing'

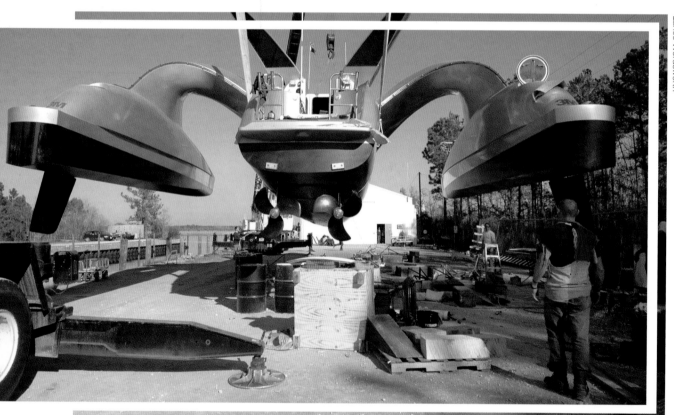

Lance Wordsworth

Craning *Earthrace* back into the water. Note the unusual-shaped carbon propellers. These were fantastically efficient in relation to fuel burn.

needed cash injection. Biodiesel and Fuels de Puerto Rico, who have hosted us here, also sign on with fuel for the first two legs of the race.

From there we head off to Barbados where we get into final race preparations. It's the night before we start and there are still a dozen projects left to complete. 'We might not have time to finish all of these,' Anthony says to me, looking down the list.

'Let's just prioritise them. What absolutely has to be finished?'

'The toilet,' says Ryan. Interestingly, he's always the one who seems to manage to block it the most. Also on the list is the email service, fuel centrifuge, and Ryan's new fixed-mount cameras to film us going through waves. As the day grinds on, we gradually tick off the jobs, and then start the final loading.

Anthony is busy trying to fit a big red toolbox into the galley. I've noticed he's like a magpie: he collects things, and they end up on *Earthrace*. And given he's the messiest person we've ever had, this toolbox doesn't bode well. Its weight we don't need. It takes up a mountain of space. And it means he'll be tempted to take that much more junk along.

'Do we really need this?' I ask him, as he's adding another screwdriver to an already full drawer.

'Absolutely,' he replies with conviction. I look at him for a few seconds and decide to give up making a big deal about it.

At 8pm *Earthrace* is finally all loaded, and we head out to a local restaurant for what feels like our last supper. It's a beautiful warm evening, and Ryan and I decide to sit outside for a while and have a chat.

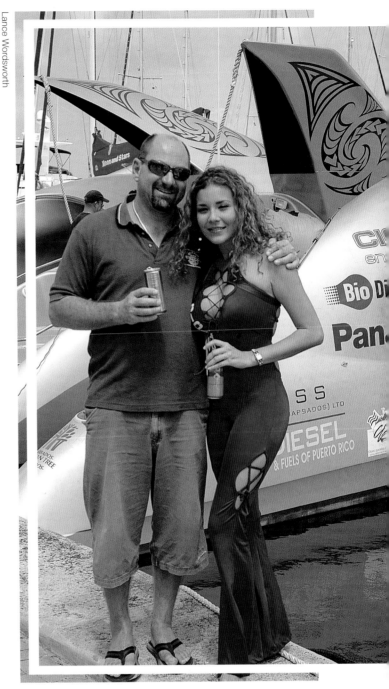

Lance Wordsworth

One of the Ciclon girls will be joining us on the last leg of the race. Not sure how suitable the spandex outfit will be but it sure looks good.

'You know, I still can't quite believe that this time tomorrow we'll actually be racing,' says Ryan.

'It's unbelievable that we managed to make it here at all.'

A group of local kids are playing soccer in the park across the road, and we can hear them yelling at each other.

'The amazing thing for me is how we pieced this together. I always thought we'd just have a few sponsors fund this, and yet it's been put together bit by bit, with literally hundreds of sponsors and people who've supported us all along the way. It's because of all this support that we're here in the first place. We're the privileged few who get the opportunity to take this boat around the globe.' Ryan takes a sip from his orange juice. 'Look at Normy in there.' I point over at Norman who is busy buying another round of drinks for us. 'He's worked like a dog for us for four days now. He

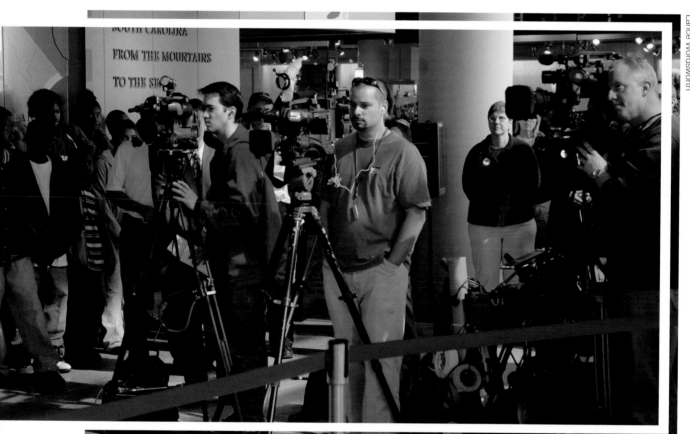

Lance Wordsworth

The press conference in Charleston with a good media turnout.

and Liza are shouting us dinner here tonight, they'll be there at the start line tomorrow cheering us on, and they'll be at the finish line when we return here in a couple of months. It's people like that who have made this all possible. And yet what do they get out of it?'

'They get my company of course,' says Ryan jokingly.

Norman comes out and hands us a drink each.

'Hey, Norman,' says Ryan, as he takes the drink. 'Why are you guys all so helpful to us here?'

Norman looks at us for a few seconds, like he's deep in thought. 'I guess 'cause I won do be involved in sumding special mon . . . and I believe in you guys.' He wanders back inside, leaving us to it.

'You know it's a bit daunting the thought of letting all these people down,' says Ryan. 'What if we don't actually get the record?'

'Look, we've already achieved what we set out to do, and that is to promote renewable fuels like biodiesel. We've had over thirty thousand Kiwis and fifty thousand Americans aboard *Earthrace*, and almost all of them will know a little about biodiesel now. We've given over a hundred TV interviews since we arrived in Vancouver seven months ago. Your footage has been seen on The History Channel, Discovery Channel, NBC, PBS, CNN and CBC. We've connected with millions and millions of people as it is, so we've already achieved what we set out to do. From here, mate, all we can do is our best. If that's good enough to get the record, so be it. But all we can do is our best. And that's all our sponsors and supporters expect anyway.'

# Part two
# The race

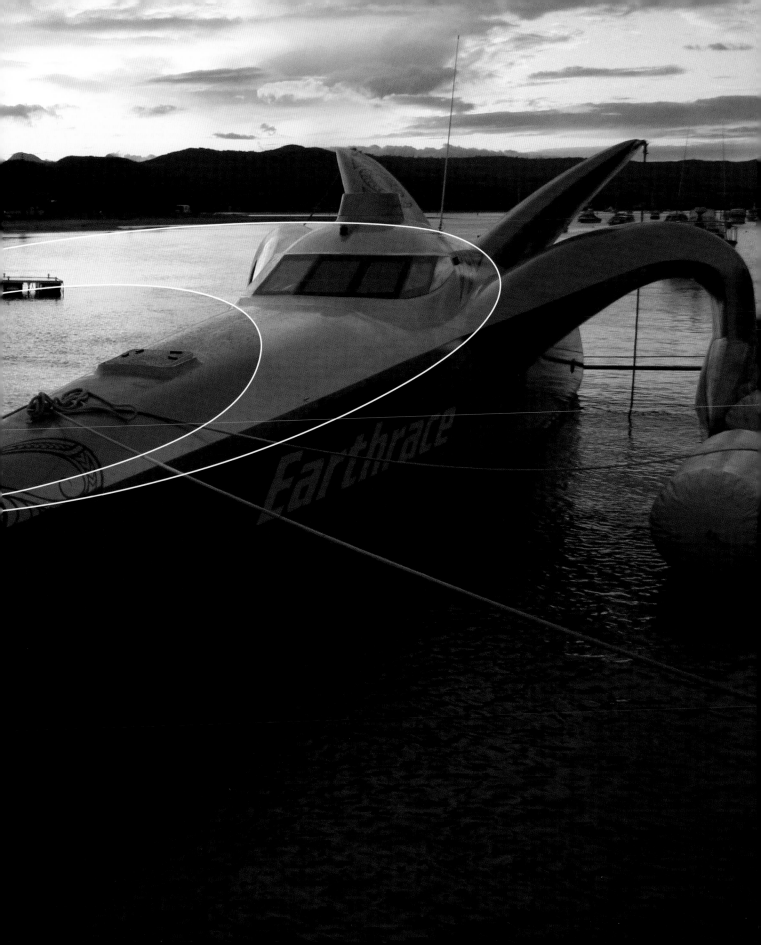

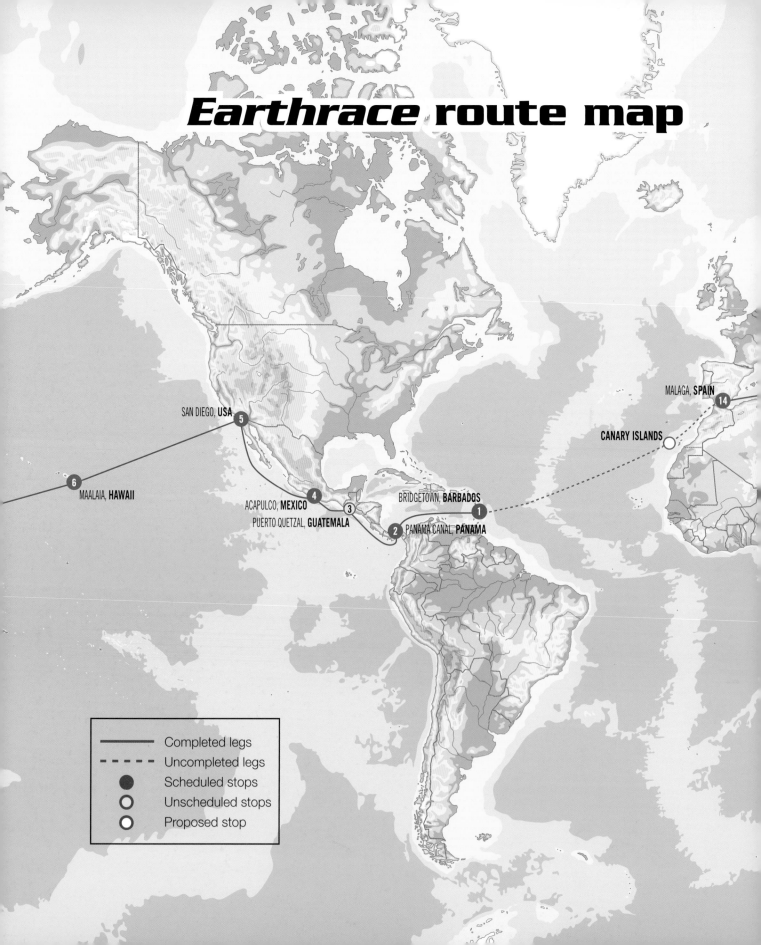

# Earthrace route map

MALAGA, **SPAIN** 14

CANARY ISLANDS ○

SAN DIEGO, **USA** 5

6 MAALAIA, **HAWAII**

BRIDGETOWN, **BARBADOS** 1

ACAPULCO, **MEXICO** 4

3

PUERTO QUETZAL, **GUATEMALA**

2 PANAMA CANAL, **PANAMA**

___ Completed legs
--- Uncompleted legs
● Scheduled stops
○ Unscheduled stops
○ Proposed stop

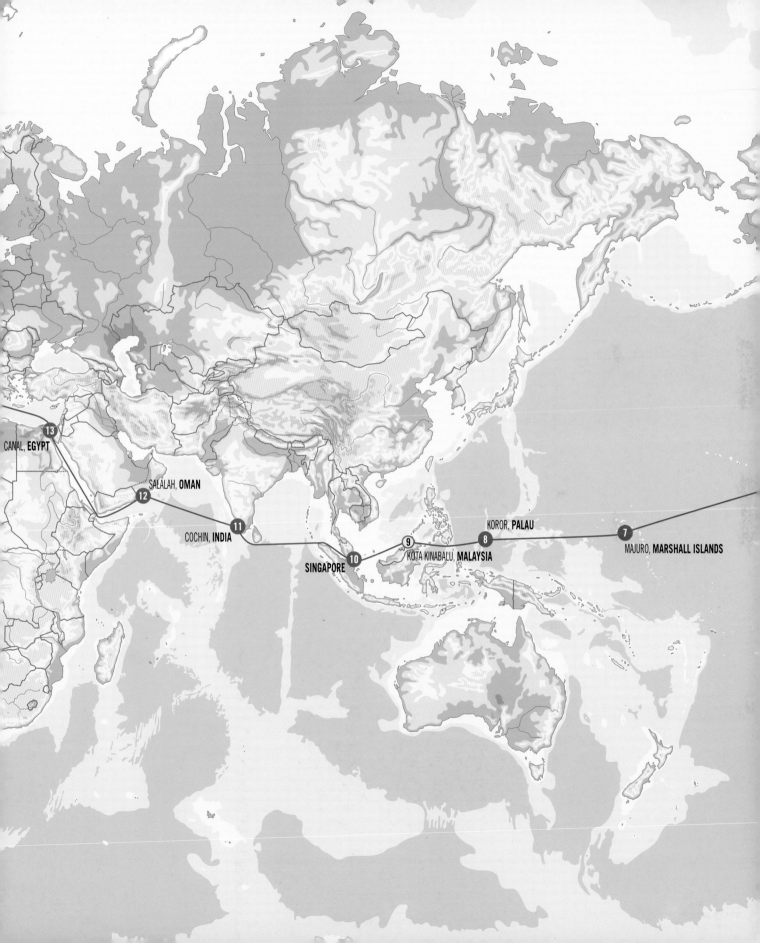

CANAL, **EGYPT** ⑬

SALALAH, **OMAN**
⑫

COCHIN, **INDIA** ⑪

**SINGAPORE** ⑩

⑨

KOTA KINABALU, **MALAYSIA**

KOROR, **PALAU** ⑧

MAJURO, **MARSHALL ISLANDS** ⑦

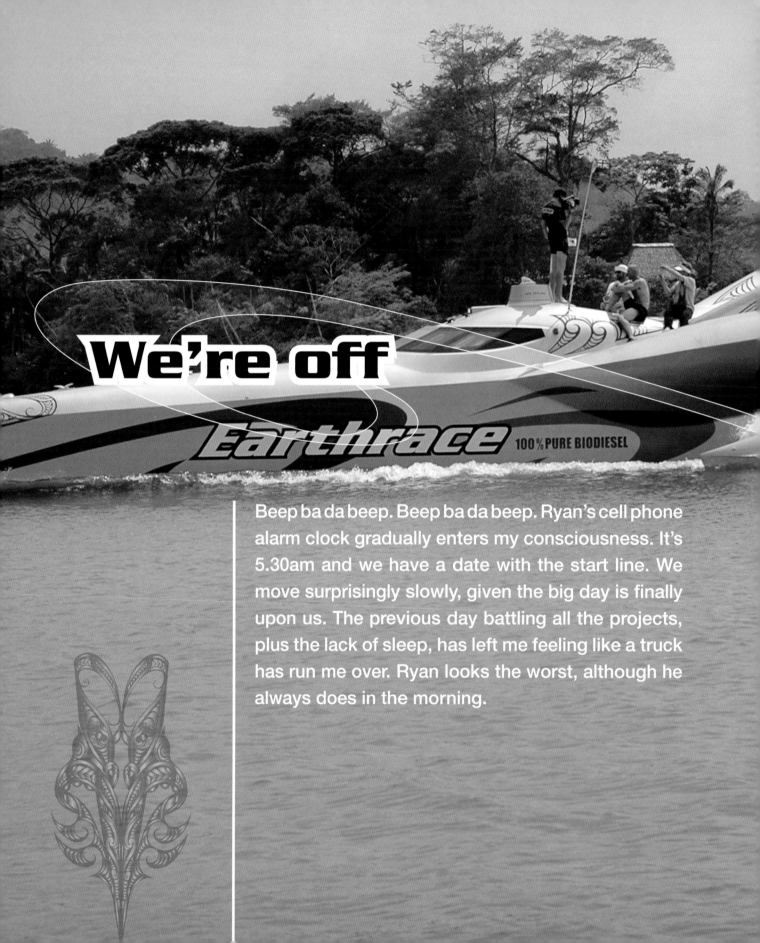

# We're off

**Earthrace** 100% PURE BIODIESEL

Beep ba da beep. Beep ba da beep. Ryan's cell phone alarm clock gradually enters my consciousness. It's 5.30am and we have a date with the start line. We move surprisingly slowly, given the big day is finally upon us. The previous day battling all the projects, plus the lack of sleep, has left me feeling like a truck has run me over. Ryan looks the worst, although he always does in the morning.

It's just after 7am as we idle into the Inner Careenage in Bridgetown, Barbados, waiting on the official timekeepers. There's a crowd of locals and tourists there to see us off, many of them waving little banners and placards. We then get a message that one of the timekeepers has slept in, and won't be in for half an hour. It turns into an hour before he appears, sauntering along the dock. Then the buoys that mark the start are still to be set, but they've disappeared. There are people jumping on and off the start boat arguing and shouting, while we're left manoeuvring *Earthrace* in the tight confines of the careenage. The boat lurches backwards and forwards and twists as we keep her in place, battling the wind and current. It's like she wants to be out of here. We all do.

Our schedule to Panama is tight as it is, and if we're late, we spend an extra day waiting for the next canal opening. So I start blabbering on the radio. 'I don't care about the yellow buoys, we'll use the two orange marker buoys outside the careenage. Just get the starters out there and we're off.' A few minutes later and the little start boat disappears out to the revised start line.

# I put *Earthrace* into gear and the engines throw out a throaty roar. We rocket past the start line

We sit there for one last minute and savour the moment. It's taken millions of dollars, thousands of hours of work and hundreds of volunteers to get us here, and finally the start has arrived. I'm a mixture of emotions: excitement at finally being here, and trepidation at what lies ahead. 'Let's roll,' yells Ryan from the roof.

I put *Earthrace* into gear and the engines throw out a throaty roar. We rocket past the start line. A Barbados flag is dropped in the water. The lads all yell and scream. We're out of here! A few boats tag along but get battered by the waves and fall away. *Earthrace* cuts silently through them, effortlessly peeling them apart. Half an hour later and the ocean is ours. Just 24,000 nautical miles to go.

'Did you feel that?' Anthony, our American engineer, yells from the cockpit. A strong vibration came shuddering up the hull. I had, but I'm not sure what it was. 'Maybe a rope or something catching the props,' I suggest. 'Or cavitation perhaps?' We concentrate, but the vibration doesn't come back. *Earthrace* at 2500 rpm is an intimidating beast. The noise is incredible. We're all wearing earplugs and noise-cancelling headphones, but the sound still gets through. There's a constant shudder that works its way along the carbon shell and into your body, and you can't escape it. It just nags at you incessantly.

We're just tucking into our first dinner on the race when Anthony comes running in from the engine room. 'The port engine filter is leaking oil.' We go down and see a pool of oil in the bilge, and the telltale black liquid dripping off the housing. Oil is like blood. You lose it and the engine dies. We turn off the engine, but then struggle to remove the filter. It doesn't want to turn. I try to unscrew it with the tool, but my arms keep getting scorched

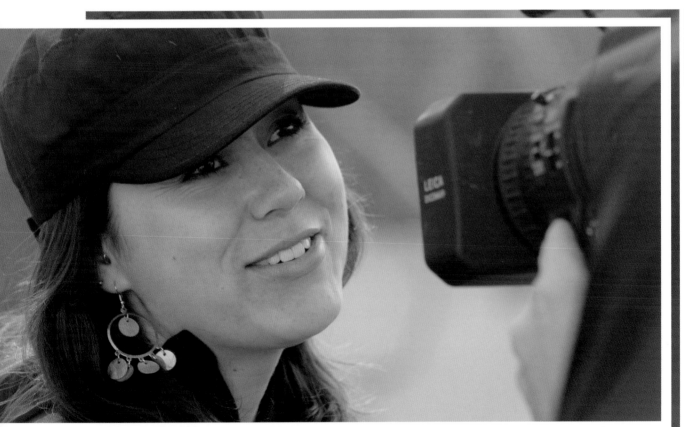

Lance Wordsworth

Devann doing a piece to camera. She got really good at handling media.

on the starboard engine, still roaring along at 2500 rpm, just inches from my face. What a nightmare.

Eventually, we lever it off with a pipe wrench and replace it. Only 10 minutes lost. If that's all we lose each day I'd be more than happy. But then we look down and see the same trickle of oil down the engine. It's not leaking from the filter at all, but somewhere just above the filter. The area is obscured beneath the heat exchanger. So 10 minutes was lost but we never solved anything. Anthony slings a small bucket beneath the leak. 'It's actually not that bad,' he says. We collect the oil and in an hour it's less than half a litre. So we decide to just collect it in a bucket, and tip it back into the engine every couple of hours, as long as our oil pressure remains good.

My stomach by now is churning. Not even a day into this attempt and we're already into trouble. How are we ever going to get right around the globe I wonder? Then I spot the cause of our problems. A bunch of bananas sits partially buried in the fruit bin.

# Not even a day into this attempt and we're already into trouble

Boats and bananas go way back. Historically, on ships, crews relied on fruit to prevent scurvy, but if bananas were taken on board, the gases they release would make the other fruit ripen too quickly. So very soon there was nothing left other than rotten fruit and the crew got sick. So bananas were banned from many boats, and they've been bad luck on *Earthrace* whenever someone has been foolish enough to bring them. So I grab the bunch and sling them overboard before they can curse us any more.

'Who the hell brought bananas on board?' I yell out. Bruce sheepishly admits he was the criminal, but looks rather perplexed at the crew's attitude. 'It was just a bunch of bananas,' he explains. I tell him the banana story and he remains bemused, looking at me like I should know better. I go off to bed, hoping the bananas haven't cursed us any more.

When you've spent so much time in the one boat, you get very tuned to the noises and vibrations it makes. It's 3am and I wake with a sense that something is not right. I lie on one arm for a few minutes and feel a constant vibration coming through, which is always there on *Earthrace*, only now it's stronger than normal.

I scurry out of bed. Bruce is driving with Anthony beside him. It feels like a problem with the propellers. The engine parameters all look OK, but the frequency is low, like a blade may be out of balance. Bruce takes *Earthrace* out of gear, and we head out to the transom step. The water is black and uninviting, as I drop in and swim underneath the stern. The light from my torch bounces off the reflective driveshafts, and there's a silent eeriness that is unnerving.

Clinging onto the driveshaft, I start looking over the propellers, and am horrified to see gouges out of the leading edge of all six carbon blades. More alarmingly, the entire face of one blade has delaminated, exposing a layer of raw carbon. 'They're totally stuffed,' I say to the lads, as I clamber back on board the transom of *Earthrace*.

I'm really worried we might not make Panama now as these propellers continue to deteriorate. The starboard prop is worse, so we drop starboard engine speed down to 1000 rpm, and crank the port engine to 1500 rpm. It's a fine line to tread. Too much grunt and we'll shatter a blade to bits, too little and the record is lost to us. The fantastic efficiency of these props was supposed to give us an edge, but instead their unreliability has cost us dearly.

We head back inside and I grab the sat phone, calling Allison who by now is with the ground crew in Panama waiting for us. Her voice is distant and delayed over the dodgy connection, but she kicks into gear once she realises our predicament. 'Can you make Panama?' she asks calmly. Her confident voice is reassuring.

'Most probably,' I reply, 'but we won't arrive until Tuesday.'

'Well,' she says, 'we'll need the existing prop and shaft details and we'll find a new set.' Getting the details is easy. Finding new props won't be, especially on a weekend.

For the next four hours there are emails and phone calls as we work through the details. Finally, it seems like the ground crew have everything they need from us, so I settle back in the driver's seat. I'm tired, but I know I'll struggle to sleep, so I may as well just drive for a while. Ryan is the same. He's sitting in the navigator's chair with an anxious look on his face.

I look down at the radar clock and realise we've been going for 24 hours. The first day has passed and we've done 590 nautical miles, which is 254 miles ahead of the existing record holder. Of course, now we're going so slowly that in another couple of days we'll be behind the old record time.

It's late in the afternoon and an email arrives from Allison. There is a prop set in Fort Lauderdale that will work, but they need machining, while there's a second possible set in California. They're a great team Scott and Allison, I think as I close the email program. The incessant vibration of deteriorating propellers, though, keeps nagging at me, so I jump up on the roof and settle down on a beanbag, trying to take my mind off it.

A pod of dolphins comes racing over to join us, leaping out as they head for our bow. They're really small, almost like the Hector's dolphins back in New Zealand. Normally, they only stay with *Earthrace* for a minute or two. We're either too fast for them, or our bow wave is so small that they lose interest. But these ones hang around for about 15 minutes, the odd one leaping out of the water in an agile display of acrobatics, which briefly takes my mind away from our problems. Another hour and it's dark, so I head back inside.

## 'Something just flashed past the windscreen. It's the third one I've seen in the last half hour'

'Oh, did you see that?' yells Paul excitedly.

'Did I see what?' I reply.

'Something just flashed past the windscreen. It's the third one I've seen in the last half hour.'

I climb into the navigator's seat and look out and, sure enough, 10 minutes later there's a streak of light as a flying fish shoots across in front of us. Flying fish are ever present in tropical waters. We've seen many kinds since we left New Zealand in July. But these ones are more aerial than most; seemingly attracted to the lights on *Earthrace*, they come flashing in arcs in front of us, catching the light as they pass.

In the morning we see the result. 'Hey, check these out,' says Anthony from the cockpit. Four tiny flying fish lie on the deck, having landed there during the night. 'How about a cook-up?' I suggest. Bruce is unimpressed, but Ryan thinks it'll make good footage. I get the knife out and have a go at filleting. They're so tiny that they just get messy. I give up on the two smallest, and am left with four tiny fillets from the two larger fish. Into the skillet they go with the skin still on with a wee dab of butter and 30 seconds later they're done. No one seems keen on being first to try them. So

I give it a go. And it is good — unbelievably good in fact. Bruce looks at us from the beanbag and turns his nose up. 'No thanks guys,' he says. Ryan has one. 'Bloody great!' he gushes. Anthony downs his. A big smile comes across his face. 'Ye of little faith,' I say to them. I quickly wolf down the last fillet before Paul smells something cooking. What a great way to start the day.

The beautiful following sea that greeted us when we left Barbados continues. Waves come rolling in from behind and the stern of *Earthrace* gets picked up. Speed starts lifting from 12 knots, sometimes getting as high as 18 knots as we surf the wave. The slender bow dips into the wave trough, cleaving apart a narrow channel. The churn of cavitation as our damaged props spin in the foamy water reminds us we're on borrowed time right now. We then drop back down the back of the wave and the cycle starts again.

Meanwhile, back on land, Scott and Allison continue their relentless pursuit of propellers. 'We think we'll get the new set the day after you arrive here,' Allison says to me over the sat phone, 'which is not perfect, but it's the best we can do.' From there we'll need to remove the old set of props, install the new set, then get the next crossing through the canal. Lots to do I realise. I look down at the GPS. We're now about 50 miles off the coast of Colombia — probably a safe distance from any pirates lurking around. My mind wanders back to when the Colombian navy shot at us last year. Wouldn't it be ironic if we met them again?

'Man that felt weird,' Anthony says to me. I'm trying to listen to my iPod and it seems as soon as the headphones go on, everyone wants to talk to you — but I did feel it too. The waves have been building steadily over the last few hours, along with the wind, and now, instead of coming from directly behind, they are coming from the sides as well.

'These waves are getting a bit gnarly,' I say. *Earthrace* normally handles a following sea beautifully, but with our props disintegrating, we're travelling so slowly that there is not much water over the rudders to control her. We're also putting most of the drive through the port engine, and this tends to skew *Earthrace* to the side, which all means we are not handling these big waves well. Every so often a wave comes through that lifts us up from the side. It is very unnerving . . . and looking around, everyone seems a little anxious.

'Let's drive her manually for a bit,' I say. Anthony flicks off the autopilot and takes control with the steering wheel. The next big wave builds from behind, sucking our starboard side in. Before we get lifted from the side, Anthony deftly flicks a quick half turn to port and it lines our stern up directly with the wave. It picks up the stern and in a few seconds we are surfing. Engine loads drop right off and we're rocking down at 18 knots. The bow buries in the wave trough and a strong whooshing noise emanates through the carbon hull. Eventually, the wave dies and we fall off the back, but not before we've had a free ride for a few hundred metres.

It is much safer than relying on the autopilot, and there's always the challenge of who the best surfer is: '20.7 knots,' Anthony yells out. It is the highest speed today. But nowhere near the 27.9 knots we clocked up in a storm back in June. Bruce settles back down in his beanbag, while Anthony lines up the next wave.

Dinner is ready and Ryan hands a plate of soup and bread down to Bruce,

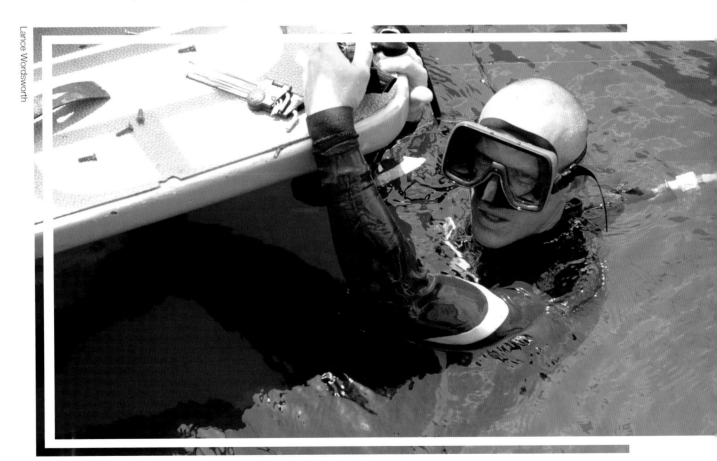

Lance Wordsworth

Changing propellers in the croc-infested waters of Panama.

by now lying prostrate on his beanbag. 'Is that it?' barks Bruce indignantly. 'What about the banquet I cooked up on Saturday?'

'Well, ya don't have to eat it,' Ryan says. Ryan looks at the thick concoction, and realises he's forgotten to add the milk. He takes the plate off Bruce and a few minutes later hands it over again, this time looking a little creamier and less like it needs a fork to be eaten.

I settle back to my iPod and soup. I'm listening to *Conscious Roots 3*, a great compilation of reggae and dub music from New Zealand. The song 'Get up' plays — my favourite track right now. My eldest daughter Danielle is 12 today, and we bought her an iPod nano for her birthday. I write her an email suggesting I can load some Conscious Roots on it for her if she likes, which of course she wouldn't like. But she's an awesome kid despite her errant taste in music.

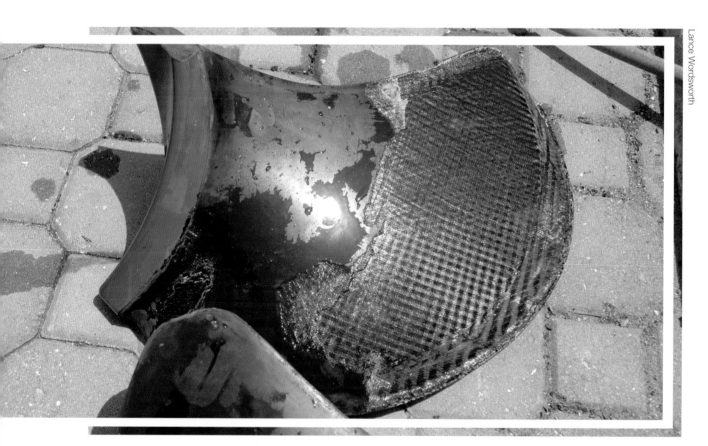

One of the damaged carbon propeller blades. Note the face has delaminated, exposing raw carbon.

The rest of the voyage to Panama goes smoothly, and we arrive there keen for a fast turnaround. The immediate job is to remove the existing propellers. I'm decidedly uneasy jumping into the water beneath *Earthrace*. 'No dive. Crocodiles,' a local had warned us a few minutes earlier, a stern look on his face as he gestured a set of jaws with his arms. Not that we have much choice. We've got half a day to pull the propellers, a job that took us three days in Barbados just a week earlier. I pull on my Orca wetsuit, kidding myself that if a croc did have a crack at me, it'd provide a little protection.

# A shadow drifts over me and I'm suddenly gripped with intense fear

Five minutes later and I'm dropping into murky dark waters, the local muttering under his breath and shaking his head in bewilderment as he saunters off. The water is shallow here. There are only a few feet beneath the props, which is good, because it allows me to stand and work with the air regulator in my mouth.

A shadow drifts over me and I'm suddenly gripped with intense fear. For a split second I think I'm about to be eaten, but I look up to see it's only Scott passing down the impact hammer. 'You're being irrational,' I keep reminding myself, as I line the hammer up on our port prop shaft. I pull the trigger and 1000 foot-pounds of torque suddenly heaves through the tool in a series of bursts. The area around me erupts in a mountain of bubbles, and my chest vibrates as the hammer wrestles with the first nut. I'm thinking it's a wicked piece of hardware, and feeling a lot easier about crocodiles. There's no way they'd be game enough to come near me with this thing thumping away. Twenty minutes later and the last of the four nuts is handed up to Scott.

'Thank God they held together long enough to get you to Panama,' says Scott. The super-high-tech carbon blades now lie like dead carcasses on the dock, the crew eying them suspiciously. 'Man, are they stuffed,' says Anthony, poking at one with his foot.

We're now just waiting on the new props to arrive. They're on a connecting FedEx flight somewhere between New Orleans and Panama. 'If we pull a small miracle with FedEx and Customs, we'll get them tonight,' says Allison. This will have us installing them in the dark, and hopefully ready for an early canal crossing in the morning. We need a miracle indeed.

A Discovery Channel crew from Canada is here for their live interview. We're juggling several TV and media crews along with all the maintenance, and it is a hectic mix throughout the day. Five o'clock rolls by and we get word that our props have been rerouted to Colombia instead of Panama. Allison is ropeable. She grabs the phone and stalks off into the yacht club with it held to her ear. At 9pm she emerges with a big smile on her face. 'You see, miracles do happen. Our props have arrived in Customs, and the Panamanian President has requested that airport staff clear them immediately for us.' At 10pm they're loaded into a truck, and just after midnight they arrive at our dock in Colon.

'Check out the pitch on these babies,' Scott comments as we lift the first prop out of its crate. Scott likes them. There was much debate over what props to use. In the end he and Allison sought the opinions of four experts before deciding on these ones. Although, interestingly, none of the experts agreed on what props we should run.

Scott and I grab the wetsuits and start installing them. By 1am we start up the impact hammer to lock home the nuts on the first one, and I'm feeling a little safer with our croc-scaring device back in action. The second prop does not seat home completely like the first. 'There's a couple of thou clearance on this,' says Scott, looking worried. We crank the impact hammer up a few more times and it improves a little, but still not 100 per cent. 'I reckon there's enough there to hold,' I say. It worries me, though, and I know it'll play on my mind for ages, but we have a canal to catch. It's 3am and we're all scurrying off to bed for a few hours' sleep, totally exhausted.

It's 6am and Anthony, surprisingly chipper for someone who hardly slept, starts his engine checks. The rest of us begrudgingly extricate ourselves from our scratchers. At seven o'clock we throw lines to leave Shelter Bay Marina. I put *Earthrace* in gear and she lurches away from the dock. But, as we idle off, there's a high-pitch ringing sound coming from somewhere. 'Oh, that's OK,' Scott says. 'Many props make noises like that.' As engine speed increases the ringing increases in pitch and intensity, then at 1350 rpm it suddenly disappears.

'How cool is that?' says Ryan. 'Our new props sing to us to show how happy they are to be on *Earthrace*.'

We do some runs up and down the bay to get initial numbers on boat speed versus fuel consumption. We're about two knots down on the carbon propellers for the same fuel burn, I note, which is not perfect, although not unexpected. The carbon blades we'd been running are super-efficient, and while these new props are not as good efficiency wise, at least they should last the race.

At 9am our pilot for the canal crossing is dropped off. He's a big lad and struggles to fit his large bum into the narrow navigator's seat. He guides us into the first lock chamber, behind the container ship *Fortune Bright*. How appropriate, I think to myself. We tie up against a tugboat, and within minutes the water starts to churn as the massive valves are opened, filling our chamber with fresh water from the lake above. It's an intense rush as *Earthrace* is tossed around, straining against the ropes that bind us to the tugboat. Eventually, the flow subsides once the chamber is full. We then untie from the tugboat, and move cautiously into the next chamber, struggling against the ever-present wind and currents that keep pushing us to the sides. It's nerve-wracking, and all the crew are on edge.

An hour later and we emerge into the freshwater lake. The Panama Canal is one of the great constructed wonders of the world. Originally started by the French and completed by the Americans, the canal came at a heavy cost, with over 10,000 people dying during construction. However, by allowing boats to travel between the Atlantic Ocean (via the Caribbean) and the Pacific, billions and billions of dollars in transport costs and fuel are saved each year. From the Atlantic/Caribbean side,

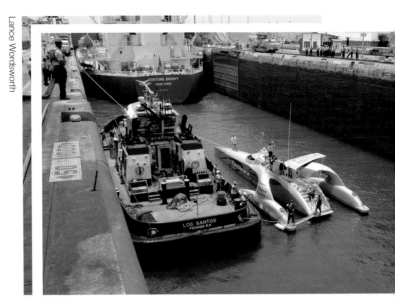

Lance Wordsworth

The Panama Canal is a truly amazing engineering feat. Here we are tying up against a tugboat before the chamber is filled. On the right-hand side are a couple of locomotives that control the big ships.

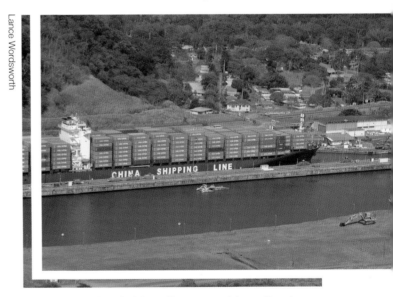

Lance Wordsworth

*Earthrace* is dwarfed by a Panamax ship as it enters into the first chamber. The Panamax ships are designed specifically to fit in the Panama Canal, and have only about half a metre clearance on each side.

you enter three chambers, each one raising you up by about eight metres. Then you go through a 30-mile freshwater lake that we're travelling on now, after which you drop down through another three chambers, to sea level in the Pacific. Quite amazing, really.

'Look over there!' yells Devann urgently, pointing at a crocodile basking in the mid-morning sun. We're passing through a narrow section of channel with lush tropical rainforest on either side of us, and most of the crew are sitting on the roof enjoying the sights. There's an amazing array of birds and wildlife on display, and even some monkeys playing in the canopy. 'You know this is one of the most amazing places I've ever seen,' Ryan says earnestly. I think back to the many wonderful places we've been privileged enough to visit: Stewart Island, Fiordland, Minerva Reef, Palmyra Atoll. They're all fantastic, and this would certainly be right up there.

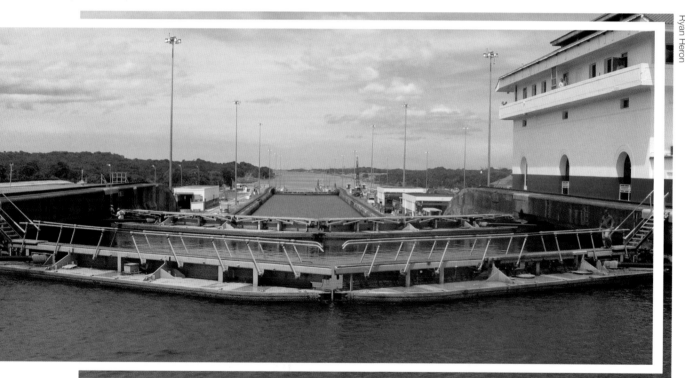

Ryan Heron

This is the view from the middle chamber looking down to sea level. The next chamber is eight metres below our current position then sea level is another eight metres below that. The filling or emptying process only takes about five minutes. Note the chamber is sealed with two sets of gates.

It's well into the evening by the time we emerge into the Pacific, weaving our way past the various container ships. Our passengers are dropped off at the famous Balboa Yacht Club then we start our journey north towards Acapulco in Mexico. 'What sort of weather are you expecting?' says Ryan. He's sitting peeling an orange and accumulating the scraps in his lap.

'Should be OK, unless we get a blow in the Tehuantepec.' This area of Mexico just north of Guatemala is notorious for massive winds suddenly gusting out of nowhere. Our plan is to approach the Tehuantepec at a distance of only 15 to 20 miles, and if the wind does get up we'll be able to sneak in close to land quickly to avoid the huge waves that will build as they head offshore. I explain the plan to Ryan, who nods his head.

# I scurry out of bed and look at the starboard engine display. It's showing low oil pressure

Our shifts during the night are two-hourly. So I'll drive for two hours then have four hours off to sleep, while Ryan and then Anthony drive. It's just towards the end of Anthony's shift when my dreams are suddenly shattered by an engine alarm. I scurry out of bed and look at the starboard engine display. It's showing low oil pressure, so we shut her down and clamber into the engine room for a look. To our horror, there's oil all over the engine and bilge. 'It's the head gasket,' Anthony says. 'Oil is leaking all around the block.' I'm not convinced, as it just seems there's oil everywhere. We refill the engine with oil and start her up. Oil squirts out a bolthole on the side of the engine. 'What does that do?' I ask Anthony, pointing to the square box that the oil is coming from.

'Not sure, bro.'

The manuals are out and it turns out to be a heat exchanger that cools the engine oil. We start to remove it, but the job just snowballs. To get the device off, we must first remove lots of other parts. The engine room is hot and loud, and the engine we're working on continues to burn our hands for hours as we remove parts bit by bit. We're continuing on with one engine so as not to lose too much time, but the motion makes even small jobs a mission. Eventually the device is off. It must be the gasket, we're thinking, although it looks OK. I'm just looking around the hole and notice a tiny hairline crack. 'There it is,' I say to Anthony.

I clean the housing up and sand away around the crack, while Anthony prepares a two-part product called JB Weld. We apply this around the crack and hole, hoping it will seal. We get the housing and engine back together then clamber forward into the helm, glad to be out of the hot and sticky engine bay. 'How long does that JB Weld take to cure?' I ask Anthony. He picks up the pack and looks at the instructions for a few minutes.

'Fifteen to 24 hours, depending on temperature.'

It's at least 45°C in the engine room now, so we decide we'll leave it for the minimum 15 hours before restarting the engine.

I look out towards Costa Rica, and there's an amazing electrical storm in full swing. Lightning streaks across the sky in a series of brilliant flashes, reminding us we're in an area that has some of the world's biggest electrical storms. We're well away from the action, though, and the seas here are dead flat. *Earthrace* is cruising along at 15 knots on one engine and seems quite happy.

The green email light flashes on, telling us a new email has arrived. Anthony opens it. 'Hey, it's from Allison. She says 50-knot winds and 15-foot seas are now predicted in the Tehuantepec, and she's recommending we go right in close to shore.' I look down at the GPS. Still a way to go to Mexico. We'll just work our way in gradually as we approach Mexico. I've always been wary of travelling close to land, as you're much more likely to get caught up in lobster pots or marker buoys, or hit marine debris. Give me 50 miles offshore any day I think to myself. But the forecast does look bad. And the closer we get to shore the lower the waves will be.

The starboard engine is restarted, and the leak, while greatly reduced, is still there. 'The crack has propagated,' Anthony says in disgust. We pull it all to bits again and apply another batch of JB Weld, this time drilling a hole at the end of the crack in the hope that it'll stop it from advancing further. Another wait of 15 hours: at this rate we'll be in Acapulco before we fix it, I'm thinking. Ground crew already have a new housing waiting for us in Mexico anyway, so if this attempt doesn't fix the leak, we may as well just finish the leg on one engine.

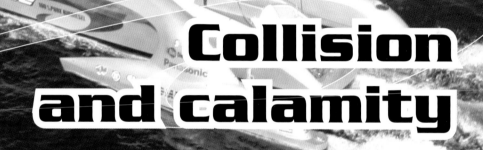

# Collision and calamity

'Where's all our food gone?' Ryan demands. This gets everyone's attention, unlike the crack in the engine, which now seems like Groundhog Day. We're missing a pile of food, but most notably some croissants and pastry that were, prior to leaving Panama, in the galley. 'I was looking forward to those,' says Ryan. I never even knew we had them, but right now they'd be fantastic. It seems no one onboard ate them at all. 'Well, they must have been stolen,' says Ryan. We ponder this a moment. Who would be wicked enough to take delicacies from a boat before it heads offshore?

We all suddenly realise who it'd be. John, the only guy we've ever met who can actually eat food in his sleep. Right now he's probably sitting in a pastry shop in California somewhere, his nimble little fingers placing delicate morsels into his eager mouth.

The lads head off to bed cursing John, while I stay up for the 10 till midnight shift, with just my iPod for company. It's a jet-black night with clear skies and a lazy half-metre swell rolling in. Two minutes before midnight. Anthony is lying asleep. I can see from the faint red glow of our LED lights his nose is bent sideways onto his pillow. I think it'd make a funny photo. I gently rock his shoulder to wake him up for his turn at the wheel.

Minutes later and I'm in my scratcher and drifting off to sleep. It's been a long day trying to repair the heat exchanger and with absolutely no success. We're now about 15 miles off the coast of Guatemala and heading towards Mexico. Ryan is struggling to sleep. He's been tossing and turning and finally decides to get up for a few minutes. He has a leak out the back, says a few quick words to Anthony, then he's back in his scratcher, trying to drift off. Anthony settles down at the controls, the autopilot gently tweaking the rudders to keep us heading north.

# We are all woken by a deafening series of crashes. I know instantly we've collided with something

Suddenly, we are all woken by a deafening series of crashes. I know instantly we've collided with something, and run out to see what's happened. Anthony is already in the cockpit area. What lies behind is like a scene from a horror movie. We've driven right over the top of a 26-foot fibreglass fishing skiff, and its tattered remains lie scattered around us. We can hear moans and yelling in the water.

One of the fishermen, 21-year-old Carlos Contreras Cruz, emerges out of the darkness and clambers onto the transom step, collapsing in a heap. A second older fisherman, Pedro Salazar Gonzalez, is wheezing and gasping for air, struggling as he bashes under the skiff remains. I jump in the water and grab his pants, hauling him up to the transom. He's limp and hardly helping himself, and I'm wondering why he doesn't just climb out. Anthony grabs his right arm and the man cries out in pain. Anthony yanks and I pull and he's unceremoniously dumped in a heap on the cockpit floor. He lies there groaning in agony.

'There's a third man in the water!' yells Anthony desperately. I'd heard him behind the starboard sponson seconds before I jumped in the water, but I'm not sure if he was the old man we'd just pulled from the water. Swimming over there I start grabbing at anything in the water. There is floating debris everywhere, including the blue buoy Anthony had hurled to the fisherman to grab on to. My hand briefly touches something fabric-like. I stop and grope in the water, but it's only a rag. My swim circle gets larger as I work away from the place I know the fisherman had been a few minutes earlier. A sense of helplessness creeps over me. There's the stench of petrol and a slick of oily fuel lies on the surface — and marine carnage all around us.

Clambering back onto the stern of *Earthrace* I get my first good look at the two fishermen. They are sitting in the cockpit, clearly in shock, blood dripping from Gonzalez's head and feet. They are shivering and looking down, seemingly exhausted. 'Let's circle the area with the spotlight!' I yell at Anthony as I run inside to start the port engine. We commence a series of slow circles through the area, dodging petrol cans, ropes and the skiff carcass, now with just a few inches of fibreglass protruding above the water.

'Over there!' shouts Ryan. I can see the spotlight flickering on a shape in the dark water. A glimmer of hope, only to be extinguished as we get closer and see it's just a sack.

We place a series of Mayday calls on VHF Channel 16. No replies anywhere. We pull Cruz into the helm and have him request help in Spanish on their local channels, but again no replies.

There are three fishing boats in a group huddled just over a mile from our position, so we decide to go and get their help with the search. I increase engine speed and there's a sudden series of shudders through the carbon hull. Ryan has a confused look on his face. 'Probably a damaged prop or bent shaft,' I say. At 800 rpm we seem to be OK, so we just creep over towards the three lights.

Cruz by now has perked up, and he's on the roof. Once we reach the boats he starts yelling at them. David, a qualified doctor who joined us for the leg from Panama to Acapulco, climbs up on the roof. His Spanish is reasonable and he starts asking them to help in the search as well. We think they're joining us but as we idle back to the collision scene, I realise they're remaining fishing. 'They just don't want to get involved,' says David to me, a look of resignation on his face. I'm amazed at this. A local fisherman lies dead or drowning just a mile from where they are, and yet they're unprepared to help.

Having failed to get any response locally, we start calling anyone who we think might be able to help. The US Coastguard, US Consulate, friends, anyone we think might be able to chase up some local support.

We track back to the Man Overboard Mark on our GPS. The skiff lies there forlornly among the debris, its outboard motor now almost submerged. 'The crap is still all here,' comments Ryan. In fact it has hardly moved at all, maybe only a few hundred metres from the original collision site. A couple of sharks are cruising around, drawn here by bait and dead fish.

## 'Tell him in Spanish that if his mate does not get the fluid now, he will die tonight'

Gonzales meanwhile has deteriorated. His blood pressure started at 104/60, but this has been steadily decreasing. David comes into the helm looking alarmed. 'It's down to 84 over 60 and still dropping,' he says with some urgency. 'Let's give him some saline solution,' I suggest. David looks surprised. 'You guys have saline?'

We dig out the packets from under the helm and sling them into our sleeping quarters, now a makeshift hospital. Cruz looks alarmed. He protests in Spanish that we are not to put anything into his friend. There's a stalemate with Cruz standing protectively over Gonzalez.

I'm starting to think that the lost fisherman has drowned, and we've got a second fisherman now looking increasingly ill. So I make the decision to abandon the search and take Gonzalez to Puerto Quetzal, some 40 nautical miles south of our current position, and from there into a hospital. It's going to take us eight hours at five knots, but without any sign of a helicopter (fat chance) or a rescue vessel (possible), we may as well make a start.

David comes back into the helm. 'Blood pressure is still dropping Pete: 70 over 60, and this other guy still won't let me administer the IV.' By now I've had enough. 'Tell him in Spanish that if his mate does not get the fluid now, he will die tonight. If he still refuses, get Ryan and Anthony to restrain him in the galley. And get the ****** saline into him!' David connects up the

IV, and clear saline fluid starts flowing into his veins. Right now his only chance at surviving this nightmare I'm thinking. Cruz looks dejected, like he has lost the battle. But he's too exhausted to fight us any more.

Gonzalez looks like he's dying. An hour ago he was lucid and talking, albeit with groans thrown in. Now he's silent, his eyes blank and looking nowhere, and his skin grey and lifeless. He's prostrate on the bunk in just his underwear, and one skinny arm hangs down. The IV fluid sits above him, cable tied to the pipe cot. Ryan and I glance down at the poor figure. We both know he's dying and in desperate need of a hospital.

I grab the sat phone. 'One man has already died!' I yell at the US Coastguard, 'and another is about to die! You call Guatemala and get a boat out here!' Assist America gets a similar rant, then the US Consulate. It's not like our problems are really their responsibility, but we know they can help, so we keep hassling them. I even place a call to the New Zealand Consulate in Mexico, but unfortunately their office is closed for the long weekend.

Meanwhile there's a slight improvement in our friend. He's taken 500 cc of IV fluid and his blood pressure has stopped dropping. Not the increase we'd like, but at least he's not dead.

At 6.45am there's finally enough light to have a look at the props. Anthony jumps in. 'The blades are all bent,' he says. 'Chuck us a large spanner.' He tries this and comes back up. 'We need something bigger.' The big monkey wrench is slung over to him. 'I need a hand with this,' he says. 'The blades are too thick.' So the two of us clamber under the stern, struggling away to straighten the props. We make a small improvement. But only just. Engine speed can be inched up a little, allowing us seven knots.

But it's unbearably slow. The problem is our starboard engine is still inoperable because of the oil leak from the day before. We're on one engine only. 'Let's see if we can keep the starboard engine going!' I yell at Anthony. My plan is to have all our spare engine oil ready to go in. We place a drip tray under the leak, and just keep recycling the fluid. So as the starboard engine loses fluid, we'll just top it up. Anthony looks dubious. He's seen the leak and knows it'll have oil everywhere in the engine room.

Five minutes later and he's ready to go. The starboard engine roars into life and I kick *Earthrace* into gear immediately, making use of the engine while we can. 'Pissing oil everywhere Pete,' comes a muffled cry from Anthony. 'Just keep her topped up!' I yell back. I'm watching the oil pressure, hovering around 3.8 bar which is normal. We might be losing fluid, but it's not affecting pressure that much. We're up to 14 knots; not great, but better than seven. It will cut our travel time in half if we can maintain this.

'Shut her down, shut her down!' screams Anthony. We grind back to seven knots and things go quiet. I poke my nose in the engine room. Anthony's face is black, completely covered in oil, with just the whites of his eyes and his teeth showing. The entire engine bay is covered in a thin spray, and the bilge is flowing with a black slick of oil. Anthony looks dejected. 'Worth a try,' he mutters.

Gonzales by now has had 1000 cc of IV fluid, and his blood pressure has sneaked up to 80/60. David checks if he's urinated yet but he hasn't. 'The trouble is he's taken a full litre of fluid into his tiny body, and nothing has come out,' explains David 'This means he's probably got significant internal bleeding.'

## At 7.23 a third email, saying a Guatemalan navy vessel has just left San Jose to meet us

Just before seven o'clock and an email arrives, saying that local authorities have been alerted, but no assets are available to help. Another series of ranting phone calls goes out. At 7.20 another email comes through. A US lieutenant-colonel has notified the local Coastguard and they are considering whether they can assist us. Then at 7.23 a third email, saying a Guatemalan navy vessel has just left San Jose to meet us. Suddenly we're not entirely alone.

Gradually, Gonzalez comes back to life. His blood pressure sneaks up. Then he's awake again, albeit a bit drowsy. Next he wants to take a pee. Not surprising when he's had 2500 cc of saline. His urine is clear. All good signs. We know he's not out of danger yet, but he's got a fighting chance at least.

Gonzalez is loaded into one of our pipe cots and made ready for transfer. Every movement causes him to wince in pain. 'Should we give him a shot of morphine?' Ryan suggests, but David feels we're better off having him alert rather than drugged up.

At 9.40am the navy vessel arrives. And then — surprise, surprise — one of the fishing boats from last night turns up. The skipper stands belligerently on the bow of the skiff, ordering his crew around. I glare down at this guy now offering his assistance. Clearly the skiff is the best option, as the navy vessel looks old and slow. A pity the fisherman wasn't so generous last night I'm thinking. There's considerable debate in Spanish on the stern over how to get him onto the skiff, while Gonzalez lies in the cockpit groaning. Finally, we manage to get him off and, seconds later, the skiff is zooming towards port, now just 14 miles away.

The navy captain then comes aboard *Earthrace*. He wants to know what happened. So I tell him the story of the most horrifying night of my life. We struggle over some of the words, and we're nearly to port before I finish. The captain came with another young man, who is surprisingly out of uniform. 'Who is this?' I ask, pointing at him.

'It is the son of the man who is now missing, and he was fishing on the boat

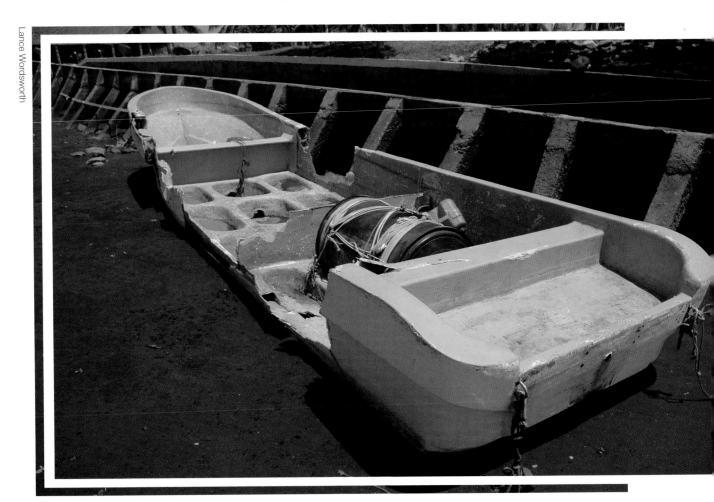

Lance Wordsworth

The damaged eight metres fishing skiff. *Earthrace* basically drove over the top of it.

last night when you went and asked them for help.' I can see in the young man's eyes he knows we're talking about him, but he doesn't understand.

'Does he know his father has drowned?' I ask, tears now starting to well up in my eyes.

'Not yet,' the captain replies, looking away, and also struggling to contain his emotions. Tears roll down my cheeks, and the gravity of last night's events finally sink in. We continue on in silence.

'I've only got one engine,' I say finally to the captain, as we're approaching the dock. 'I might need one of your boats to give us a hand docking.' There's a stiff breeze blowing us towards the wall of Puerto Quetzal. The captain looks unimpressed, as if I should know how to dock a boat with one engine by now. I convince him to have one of his patrol vessels nearby in case we get into difficulty. They've been shadowing us for ages, I'm thinking, so we may as well have them give us a hand if we need it. But in the end *Earthrace* glides gently against the dock and the crew quickly get ropes tied, making us secure.

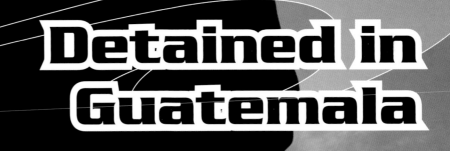

# Detained in Guatemala

We can see that word is definitely out. There's an army of military people and officials waiting for us on the dock, all looking down sternly. The scary bit for a Kiwi is all the guns. Every second person is packing a weapon of some sort, and many of them are pointed aggressively in our direction.

A roll of yellow tape comes out and, before we know it, *Earthrace* is labelled 'Crime Scene' in Spanish.

The captain gives us strict instructions. 'You may not leave this vessel tonight.'

'Are we under arrest?' I enquire. 'Yes. No. Mmm. Sort of. It is for your own protection.' I don't mind either way. I'm sure there's a procedure for them to follow through after an event like this, but I'm keen to know if I am actually under arrest, and if so, what we are charged with. In the end I let it slide.

The first of the officials make their way into the sweaty helm, which still reeks of vomit and urine. Customs, Immigration, Agriculture, shipping agent, port captain — they all come forward with their paperwork and we diligently fill out the forms. The port captain when he's finished leans forward and whispers in my ear. 'The next man is from the Ministerio Publico. Be very careful what you say to him.' I steal a glance at the man waiting next in line. He's short and solidly built, with an almost Asian look, and his face is pockmarked from acne scars.

I move forward and shake the prosecutor's hand, 'Hi, I'm the skipper. What can I do for you?'

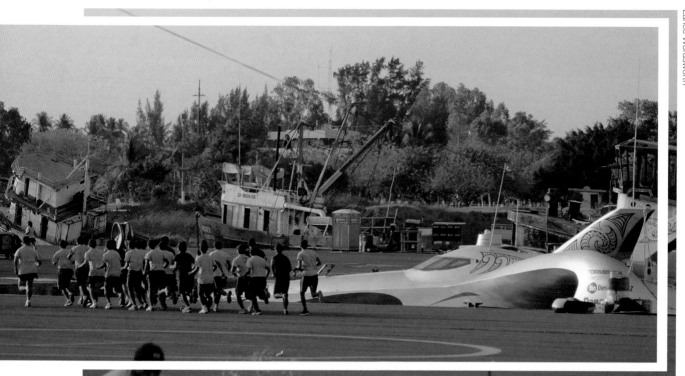

Lance Wordsworth

*Earthrace* docked at the military base in Puerto Quetzal (Guatemala). The boats in the background all have court cases pending for various offences, and some have been there for years. We didn't want to be at the end of the queue.

'We need your statement. We write now,' he says in faltering English.

'But I have no lawyer,' I say. 'Nor do I have a translator. I cannot sign anything until I have both of these.'

'We provide,' he snaps back, and he introduces us to the guy behind him. 'Who is this?'

'Umm, I'm with the Ministerio Publico and I can translate,' he says, his English with a strong American accent.

'What about an independent lawyer?'

The two guys look at each other then the translator suggests we don't really need a lawyer because all they need is a statement of what happened.

'Look, I appreciate your help here, but until I and my crew have our own translator and our own lawyer, I'm not prepared to say or sign anything.'

The prosecutor glares at me and then storms off, barking orders at one of his offsiders as he goes.

The boat seems like a haven from all the hostility outside. People are glaring menacingly down at us, but in here we feel safe. An email comes in from the ground crew. They will arrive in Guatemala tonight. We jump on the sat phone and start making phone calls. We need a lawyer and a translator sorted. Eventually, the crowd of military people dwindle off and we're left with just our military guards for the night. Four blokes with assault rifles, pacing backwards and forwards and keeping an eye on us, and a navy vessel tied off to our stern.

Ryan, Anthony and I sit in the cockpit, reflecting on the nightmare . . . and there's a question that needs answering. I can tell Anthony's expecting it. An experienced boat captain with a 100-ton licence has crashed *Earthrace* into another vessel, and it's resulted in one, possibly two deaths. How could this happen? Anthony lowers his voice, and recounts the minutes leading up to the event. 'There were three fishing boats over to port, about a mile or two away. I could see their white lights, and there was a faint blip on the radar from them. I wasn't sure initially if it was three boats or one. Next, I see a faint red flashing directly ahead, and a second later we collided. I never picked them up on radar, and I never saw any white light.'

'Well, why didn't you stop when you saw the red light?'

'There was just no time. From the moment I first saw the tiny light, to when we collided, was only a couple of seconds.' Anthony is in tears, and he's struggling.

'And you're sure there was no solid white light?'

'Absolutely,' he says, and he wipes off a couple of tears now rolling down his cheeks.

I remember when I was swimming looking for the third fisherman I'd picked up a small flashing light in the water. It was probably meant for pushbikes, with three or four LEDs in a row — hardly a marine light, and certainly not visible through 360 degrees.

'So we didn't see them until it was too late, but they probably saw us. Why do you reckon they never got out of the way?'

'Because they were all asleep,' says Ryan.

'How do you know?'

# So they had no solid white light and they were asleep, but it still doesn't explain why Anthony never picked them up on radar

'Because Cruz told me. They had set some long-lines, and were asleep drifting until it was time to check them . . . and at the time of the collision, they were still all asleep.'

So they had no solid white light and they were asleep, but it still doesn't explain why Anthony never picked them up on radar. The panga we collided with was fibreglass and with low freeboard, which would give it a relatively low radar signature, but it would still show up. We'd seen a couple early in the evening and they showed up OK. In the back of my mind, I suspect that Anthony was probably concentrating on the other three boats to port, instead of looking directly ahead, and that, combined with a dodgy flashing light and sleeping fishermen, led to the accident.

The three of us settle back to our cockpit. It's a beautiful, warm, silent night, except for the crunch of gravel under the guards' boots above us. We all realise we haven't slept or eaten in ages, and it's been an exhausting day.

'Ahoy there,' comes a familiar voice, as David arrives on the dock above us.

'Any news on Gonzalez?' I ask. David had travelled with the fisherman to hospital, and we're all anxious to know what happened.

'Well, first off,' he says, 'Gonzalez is to be operated on tonight. We're hoping he'll be OK, but we just don't know yet. Secondly, an angry mob of family members nearly lynched me today at the hospital. And, thirdly, you are requested to join Señor Munyos here at the officers' mess for dinner.' The officer standing next to David talks to the men patrolling, then motions us to climb onto the dock.

'Look Dave, I'm not really sure we should leave. The captain gave me strict orders to remain aboard *Earthrace*.' Señor Munyos makes it very plain I am being ordered to join him. He has a handgun in a holster and a stern look on his face. So we clamber up and head off to the officers' mess for a welcome meal.

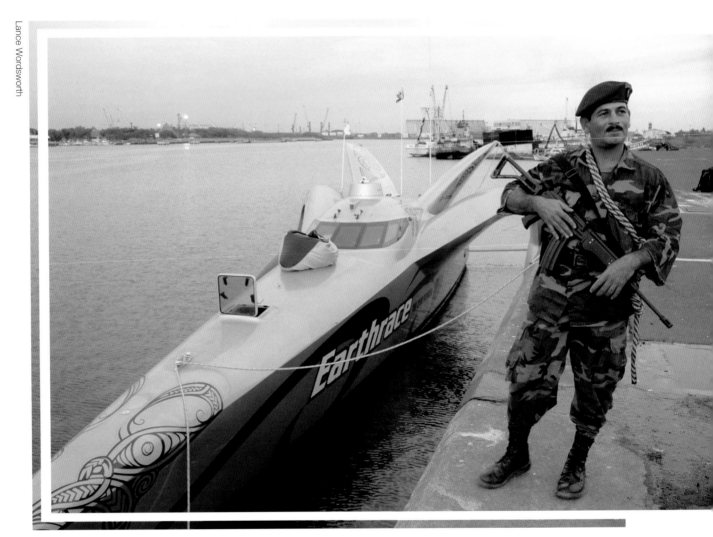

Lance Wordsworth

*Earthrace* under armed guard in Puerto Quetzal, Guatemala.

After dinner, we are ushered over to meet the commandante, apparently top dog on the base, and I'm wondering what this is all about. We walk into his office and there are Scott, Allison, Lance (a volunteer/photographer from New Zealand) and Dave, waiting for us. It's an emotional reunion. We're not alone in this, and our team has just doubled in strength, but we're going to need every one of them, I remind myself. We talk long into the night about what we need to do, and it's an exhausted crew that are finally dropped back to *Earthrace* for some sleep.

'Banana banana banana.' Spanish has a tendency to sound like this. Señor Munyos is telling us he's here to take us to breakfast. He's standing on the dock waiting for us. A big smile and a handshake greet us as we clamber up. We wander into the mess hall and there's a similarly warm reception. I'm a little surprised, because last night, especially on the dock, our reception wasn't exactly welcoming.

# 'What happened is an accident that could happen to any seamen'

I'm ushered to a seat next to the port captain. 'What do people here think of us?' I enquire. 'Well,' he says, 'when you arrive, we only know one story. But last night we learn your side of the story, and we know you did everything you could. And you saved one of our fishermen.' I wasn't sure we had saved him at all, although we did at least give him a fighting chance with the saline solution. He goes on, 'What happened is an accident that could happen to any seamen.' I'm wondering who told them our side of the story, when I see the navy captain who'd escorted *Earthrace* in the previous day talking animatedly to a group of officers, and pointing in our direction. He's the only local person I've discussed events with, but now it seems everyone knows, which is a good thing.

We'd also given copies of the *Earthrace* DVD to a few of the officials who came aboard the night before, and it seems these are now doing the rounds. As we're escorted around the base there are warm smiles and handshakes to greet us. 'Buenos dias,' many of them say. In the space of twelve hours we've gone from pariah to novelty, even if only inside the military compound.

'We here are all men of the sea.' Scott's translating the commandante's words, as we sit diligently in his office. He's a tall man, probably in his late

fifties, with a warm, generous smile. 'What happened yesterday is an accident, and I am sorry that you now find yourself here in Guatemala. Unfortunately, you are not the first boat to have such an accident. Last year we had over 30 collisions, and each time we try to get the fishermen to have lights and to wear life jackets and each time nothing changes . . . and unfortunately people here will continue to die.' He stops for a minute and looks out his window at the troops marching down below. 'My job,' he continues, looking back at us, 'is to keep you safe and to look after you. If there is anything you need, you ask.' I look back at the commandante, who is sitting there with his palms open.

'Internet?' I enquire, not really expecting a positive outcome.

The commandante gestures that I can use his computer, getting up from his desk and ushering me to his seat. Wow! How cool is that? I'm under military guard at a base, and the head honcho has given me his PC to use. Unbelievable.

'Well, what about an office to work from?' says Scott. El Commandante ushers us into a training room immediately adjacent to his office. 'Perfecto,' replies Scott. 'And I bet we can get Internet through that as well,' pointing at the RJ45 jack in the wall. Ten minutes later and we're linked up with two Internet connections, a couple of cell phones that Allison had bought on the way in, and our own room. *Earthrace* has a new base.

'Right, what needs to be done?' asks Allison, as we're busy arranging tables and chairs.

'Well, first off, let's call the hospital and find out how Gonzalez is. We should see if we can meet the fishermen and their families, and we need to finalise our lawyers. I'm not really sure what the procedure is to get us released from here, so we need to do some digging on that. We also need to get Scott down to *Earthrace* to check for damage and start on repairs.' Scott wanders out to check *Earthrace*, while Allison calls the hospital. Ryan and I both log into our email and start working through them.

'Some news on Gonzalez,' Allison says, putting her cell phone down a few minutes later. 'He was operated on last night, and had a perforated stomach, a perforated intestine, a fractured sternum, and considerable internal bleeding. The prognosis, though, is the operation went well and they expect him to recover. They also said that the saline you guys administered saved his life.' The amazing thing is we nearly didn't have saline at all. A doctor in Charleston came down and asked if we needed any medical equipment, and all I could think of at the time was saline solution.

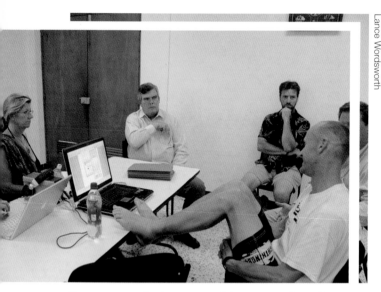

The commandante gave us this room at the military base to use. Here the insurance guys are trying to explain options to get the boat and crew released. Left to right: Allison, Guiermo (insurance representative), Scott, Fernando Lorenzo (insurance representative) and myself.

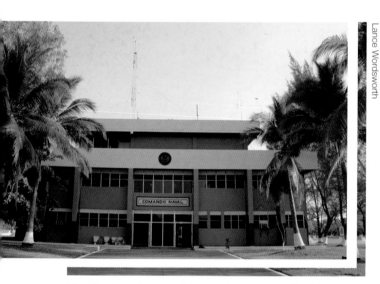

The Guatemalan naval base where we worked from. Our office was on the top floor. The commandante gave us free rein to go anywhere we liked on the base.

I go back to my laptop. There's an email from my daughter Alycia back in New Zealand. She's upset because her didgeridoo got stolen at school camp. I'm wondering if this is all worth it. I should be back at home with Sharyn and my two girls. And a fisherman wouldn't be dead and another in hospital. My mind wanders off to what seems like a lifetime ago now. We'd bought the didgeridoo in 2002 on an amazing holiday around Australia.

'Pete. The US Consulate is on the phone and they want to meet us in the morning,' says Allison. I'm brought back to reality with a thump. 'And the Ministerio Publico people are downstairs demanding a statement from you.'

The warmth of the military people towards us continues to surprise. They diligently turn up on request, driving us to the boat, the mess hall, the commandante's office, anywhere we want to go on base. One thing we're not allowed to do, though, is work on the boat, despite being forced to sleep on it. 'The guards won't let me anywhere near it,' Scott had said in disgust. At the moment we still don't know what damage there is under the hull, or how much work there is in fixing the props. But they won't even let us look. We make another request to the commandante, but he's adamant. We cannot look under the waterline.

The situation is that the Office de Publico must carry out an inspection of the vessel. But we seem unable to get them to come and perform it. I'm wondering what they hope to find. It is not like we are disputing the fact that a collision took place. We spend much of the morning hassling people but we're unable to connect with the right ones.

'How about we go and kick a rugby ball

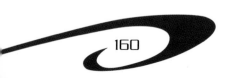

around for a while?' I suggest to Ryan. We're bored, and a run around will do us good. I grab the Waikato Chiefs rugby ball from the forward bunk and run onto the courtyard above *Earthrace*. We start passing and kicking the ball around, and one of our guards comes up. 'You play dere,' he says, pointing his rifle at a paddock behind the barracks. 'Safer.' We wander over. It's too small really, and bumpy. But we give it a go anyway. Ryan's first kick is a beautiful spiral right into the corner, and as I'm turning to chase it down, my foot dips in a hole and I crash in a heap on the ground. Searing pain burns up my leg. I look down and there's a golf ball-sized bulge sticking out from my ankle.

'Get some ice!' I shriek at Ryan, and he scampers off. I can tell at the very least it's a bad sprain, but I'm just praying it's not broken. I put some weight on my bad leg. The pain seems the same. I do a tiny hop on the bad leg and it hurts like hell, but not the searing pain you'd have from damaged bones. This is a trick I learnt in our Offshore Medic training. To tell if bones are broken or cracked, just load them by weight say, or jar them a little, like a small jump. If the bones are damaged, you'll have wicked pain. Another minute and my whole ankle has ballooned up. Right now I need ice to stop this getting worse. Ryan runs back with a couple of bottles of water. 'The medic is on his way,' he pants.

Finally, a driver arrives. It turns out he's taking us to the medic. We arrive at the Military Infermaria, the hospital, and there's no one there. 'All I want is some ice,' I yell at the driver, who clearly speaks no English. We sit down and wait, my ankle getting ever worse from the swelling. The medic arrives. He fossicks around and comes out with a solid blue ice pack, but it hardly touches any of my ankle. 'Ryan. Go in there and find some small blocks of ice,' I snap, pointing at the kitchen. Ryan disappears. I can hear him scraping at something. He comes back with a couple of fistfuls of the icy stuff you get around a freezer. Perfect. We pack it around the pregnant ankle. It hurts, but I know it helps. Just a pity it took 20 minutes to get.

I hop back to our office next to El Commandante. It's then that I first notice my shadow. A small man in Military Police uniform is following me at a distance. He walks behind buildings and trees, but always keeping me close to his field of view. I hop up to him and introduce myself. He speaks no English, and all I can get is his name is Sanchez. Then at seven o'clock he is changed for another guy.

'It's like being in a spy movie,' I say to Ryan. 'Yeah, and I could take both of them,' Ryan replies. In fact, for military police they're not the most imposing of figures. I reckon I could even escape in my current disabled state.

'Word from the lawyers, Pete. The inspection is happening now.' Allison sounds quite excited. 'And you're due in court tomorrow morning.' In fact, I was supposed to be in court today, but it was postponed. As for the inspection, that is good news. We wander — and hop — down to the boat. There's a group of people sniffing around, a couple of them with scuba gear on. They spend much of their time looking at nothing in particular, although they are especially keen on the radar and night vision system. 'Can we work on our boat now?' Scott asks the inspector after they're done. It seems there's one last bit of paper we need, and we can finally work on *Earthrace* again.

An hour later and the paperwork, complete with signatures and stamps, arrives with Scott. He throws on his wetsuit and gets to work. 'Rudders look good!' he yells out. 'Starboard sponson OK . . . port sponson some scrapes but nothing serious. Port propeller with four damaged blades . . . starboard propeller with three damaged blades.' Scott methodically works around the boat. He finally ends up near the bow and takes a long time under the water. 'There's hull damage under here,' he says, pointing beneath the ballast tank, 'but I think we can just repair it with Splashzone.' Wow. It could have been much worse.

Scott and Anthony work late into the night straightening the propellers. They're basically using a couple of sledgehammers to panelbeat them back into shape. We're not entirely sure it will work, as the props are so misshapen, but it's our best chance. We just need them good enough to get us to Mexico.

I clamber down into *Earthrace* and sit in the navigator's seat for a while thinking. Give us another day and, props permitting, the boat will be ready to leave. But when *we'll* be able to leave is another matter. Some are saying we'll be here for six months and others are saying a few days. If it does start to really drag out, the rest of the crew should be able to leave, as I'm the one responsible. There are also the fishermen's families to consider. I'd wanted to meet them but so far we've hit a blank wall. I look up at the dock and I can see my shadow keeping a watchful eye on Allison as she wanders down to see us.

'No court appearance tomorrow, Pete. They're now saying maybe Monday.' Allison gives us a quick rundown on progress, although this

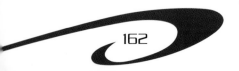

seems more like a lack of it. I've been itching to get in front of the judge and present what happened, and yet every day they delay our appearance. The good news is the lawyers are meeting with the families later today.

The law here is complicated. There is the civil side and the criminal side, and at the moment the two are tied together in a web. For us to get out of here, we must reach agreement with the families, and also satisfy the court that the collision was not our fault. But untangling the web is not that simple.

Fernando, the agent employed by our insurance company, is trying to explain this to me but I'm just getting frustrated. 'Can't we just treat the two separately?' I ask. Fernando goes off on some tangent and loses me again. 'And how come the judge keeps putting us off?' I demand. Fernando explains the judge can do whatever he likes with his day. And he can hear the cases when he likes. I'm thinking we should call the US Consulate and get them to exert some pressure. We still haven't been charged with anything, after all. Fernando goes off on another tangent. Eventually, he and his advisors leave to meet with the families, and I'm only slightly wiser on how things work here.

## I'm thinking we should call the US Consulate and get them to exert some pressure

My leg is still aching, and I hardly slept last night. It didn't seem to matter what angle I put it on. It's an ugly sight, and has started to go blue from bruising. 'You're an elephant man,' says Ryan, as I sit down at the lunch table and put my swollen leg up on a spare chair. My shadow comes past and makes a series of disapproving clucking noises. He's given up trying to be in the background now. He just walks beside me wherever I go.

We head back to our office, and everyone is talking about press releases. Until now we haven't let anything out, other than a couple of interviews back to New Zealand. Nor have we done any blogs, and everyone in the team has a strong opinion. 'There's no way we will gain anything from a press release now,' says David, 'and if any of it gets aired in Guatemala it'll just piss everyone here off.' A couple of others in the group murmur their agreement.

Another call from one of Anthony's friends then comes through. It seems his family and friends have been running a tag team to keep up the

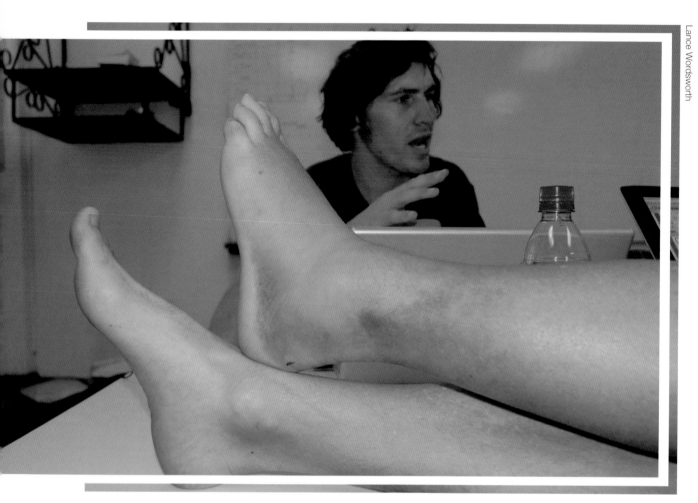

Lance Wordsworth

Ryan slinging in some ideas, with my sprained ankle looking pathetic.

pressure on us not releasing anything. I snap and tell her to stop hassling us. Next she starts telling me about what the State Department has advised her. To be fair, she and the family are only trying to give us advice, and this lady was really helpful in getting the US Consulate involved on the night of the accident. But I've spent well over an hour listening to them on the phone today and the time just isn't productive.

We're back in the office and Scott reckons we should run the press releases. Allison is on the fence. John calls in from Panama. 'We must have a press release out there Pete. We cannot hide any longer.' I wander into the spare email room we've commandeered to be alone for a bit. We've hardly achieved anything today because we're all arguing about what to release.

The thing is we have nothing to hide. It was an accident, caused in a large part by a boat not having a white light and the fishermen all being asleep. It doesn't completely excuse the fact that a collision took place, but it certainly places some of the blame on the fishermen. It would seem if we make the wrong decision, I'm the one who will cop it. As captain of the boat, I'm rightly responsible. Anthony was driving, but the Guatemalans have no interest in him, and if anyone is forced to spend time behind bars, it will be me. So, bugger it. We'll just tell the story of what happened and get it out there.

I wander back into the office. The debate has continued in my absence. 'Team,' I say, 'we are running the press release. We have nothing to hide, and it is better that people know what happened than speculate. From now on, it is up to Devann and me to determine what goes out.' David starts a sentence but I stop him. 'Look David, it's my call, and I'm going to run it.'

I grab Scott. He's written a couple of blogs but they were put on hold. 'Get them loaded Scott. From tonight, I want all blogs and press releases up to date, and that includes yours.'

Devann in San Diego is stressed. She's been getting pressure from Anthony's family not to send out the press release as well. I tell her to just do it, and she obediently starts the email server beaming our press release all over the world — and then things go ballistic. Phone calls and emails start rocking in from all corners of the globe. They want pictures, video footage, radio interviews and additional information. Devann and I are run off our feet as news agencies around the world pick up the story. It may not be the positive story we would like, but media is certainly into it.

My final job of the day involves Anthony, and I've been avoiding it all day. This guy has given his life to *Earthrace* over the last few months, but given his role in the accident I've decided I cannot continue with him as crew. He's already given this some thought. 'You know Pete,' he starts, 'it might be better if I step down as engineer.' His voice starts to falter. 'And maybe help you guys from San Diego or North Carolina.' I can't help but admire him. He's one of the most outstanding people we've had on the team, and he truly believes in what we're doing. My mind wanders back to a few days earlier when he emerged from the engine bay, his face completely covered in oil. Anthony has been a loyal servant of *Earthrace*, and has done everything I've asked. I feel like I'm letting him down by letting him go. But deep down I know it is the best for the team. We decide he'll fly home as soon as we get permission from El Commandante.

I lie awake thinking of the sacrifices people like Anthony and Devann continue to make for *Earthrace*. No one is getting paid, and yet the hours they all do are horrendous. What a strange alchemy *Earthrace* is that it can engender such commitment from people for no reward. I start to wonder if I'm asking too much of people who are overly generous. It's something I've thought about many times . . . and I still don't know the answer.

It's 10am the next day and word comes through that an agreement has been reached with the family. This is good news. Our insurance will pay to assist the family of the lost fisherman, the medical bills of the injured fisherman, and also to purchase a new fishing boat, hopefully complete with white light. The good thing with this is it does allow these families to move on from what has been a devastating tragedy. They are a desperately poor people, and the ground crew sees this every time they leave the military compound. It still has me meeting the judge on Monday, and he will make a decision on whether I'm to stand trial in their equivalent of a criminal court. Assuming he doesn't delay us again, of course.

I give Allison a call on her cell phone. 'Let's see if the family will meet us now.' We'd been trying to meet them from day one, but the lawyers had been fending us off. Now that a settlement has been reached, I'm hopeful they'll let us at least express our sorrow at what has happened. I have also been considering whether we continue with the record attempt. One man is dead and another injured in hospital because of *Earthrace*, and I'm thinking that perhaps we should abandon the record attempt altogether. It'd be good to talk these things over with the families and get their thoughts.

Scott comes wandering in with a big grin on his face. 'All crew now have permission to leave, with the exception of you,' he says, pointing a finger at me. So we can organise a flight back to the US for Anthony. I know his family will be pleased to have him out of here. 'Oh and we've finished panelbeating the propellers, so the boat is ready to test.' Scott is like a Trojan. He slings himself at jobs and continues to get them sorted. He'd be one of the most productive people I've ever worked with, and he continues to amaze me with his work rate. It means, subject to testing the props, *Earthrace* is ready to leave. Just a pity we won't be allowed to yet. I put my ankle back up on the table. 'That looks worse than ever,' says Scott, poking the bruise with his finger. It's gone a combination of blue and yellow, but at least I can put a little weight on it now.

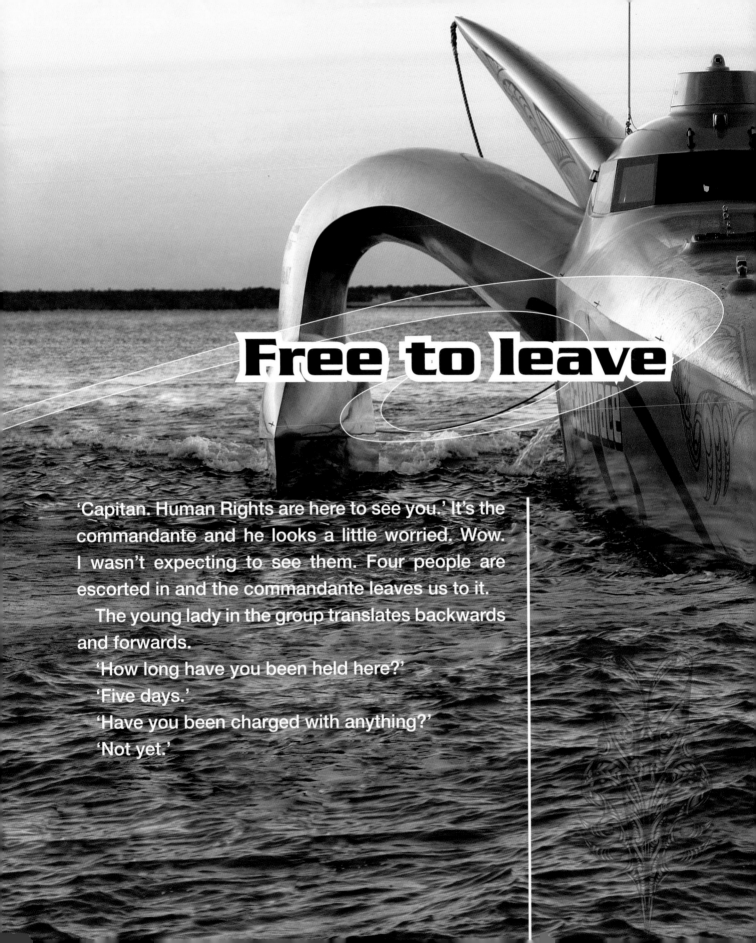

# Free to leave

'Capitan. Human Rights are here to see you.' It's the commandante and he looks a little worried. Wow. I wasn't expecting to see them. Four people are escorted in and the commandante leaves us to it.

The young lady in the group translates backwards and forwards.

'How long have you been held here?'

'Five days.'

'Have you been charged with anything?'

'Not yet.'

There's some discussion in Spanish, then the translator turns to me. 'They cannot detain you for five days without charge. There is a maximum of just 48 hours.'

Now, this is news to me. It means I've been detained illegally if they're right. What have my lawyers been up to? We call in the commandante and he explains he is simply obeying orders. We ask to see the orders, and he produces an official note from the Ministerio Publico. The Human Rights people pore over the document, and there is much debate in Spanish. 'It seems,' starts one of them, 'that this document is invalid because it has not been signed by a judge, and only a judge can request people be detained. Secondly, it can only be used for up to 48 hours before charges must be laid.'

'So that means, I can walk out of here now?' I ask.

'Yes, you can.'

# 'So that means, I can walk out of here now?'

El Commandante looks concerned and holds up his hands. 'Capitan. I am given my orders to detain you and keep you safe. This I have done. And I still have those orders.' There is more debate in Spanish, with the Human Rights people arguing that the orders are invalid. Finally, the commandante turns to me. 'Capitan. Legally you can leave this base. But I am requesting you not to. When you first arrived here, I received a call from the Minister of Defence, my boss, and he told me to ensure your safety. I then received the paper orders from Ministerio Publico with the same request. If you leave and anything happens, it will be very bad for me.'

I think about this for a short time. I'm certainly tired of being detained. While I can go anywhere on the base, there's just nothing to do. You don't realise how valuable your freedom is until it's taken from you. But if I leave now, the military, who until now have been extremely supportive of us, may suddenly withdraw their assistance. My goal is to get my crew and *Earthrace* out of here as quickly as I can, and if I annoy the commandante, it might end up costing us more time.

'Commandante,' I say, 'I will remain here, but only as a favour to you.' He shakes my hand graciously and has a relieved smile on his face.

The rest of the crew head off for a weekend in the touristy town of Antigua, leaving me alone on the boat. It's early evening when Señor

Munyos comes running down to see me, 'Capitan. Capitan. You like beer?'

'Si, si,' I reply with a silly grin on my face, and they bundle me in the back of a beat-up old Toyota. My shadow suddenly realises he's about to lose me and comes running after us, but he's too late, as Señor Munyos plants his foot and we disappear down the dusty road. I look back at the comical sight of my shadow running after the car and waving, and the officers in the car laughing at him.

We're onto our second beer before my shadow finally makes his way into the officers' bar, nestled in among the trees on the edge of the compound. He's a tiny little man, probably in his forties, and he smiles sheepishly as he sits down beside me. I pat his shoulder and offer him a beer. He steals a glance at the officers all around and declines. 'Is it OK if he has a drink?' I ask Señor Munyos. The officers have a quick debate then pass him a beer. He guzzles it down eagerly, much to the amusement of the officers, who quickly sling him another.

A few hours later and we've moved on to Ciclon and vodkas. We're down to the hard-core half dozen officers by now, and the barmaid has left, leaving the keys with us. My shadow has fallen asleep, the concoction of beer and vodkas too much for his tiny frame. We carry him out to the Toyota and dump him in the boot. 'The ratings are normally not allowed alcohol on the base,' Munyos explains, 'and so they tend to get drunk very easily.' Easily indeed, I think. We drop him at the boat to sleep off the alcohol, and the rest of us head over to the officers' quarters to finish the final two packs of beer.

The captain who had escorted us last weekend disappears, then returns and asks for quiet. 'Capitan,' he says ceremoniously, 'this is the badge I received for outstanding service in the Guatemalan navy, and I would like you to have it.' He proffers in the palms of his hands a gold badge. I'm starting to think it's just a drunken gift, because we've all had a skinful by now. The officers, however, are deathly quiet and looking at me expectantly. Man, this is too much. I start to decline and he holds up his hands for me to stop speaking. 'We here are all men of the sea. And everyone in this room has respect for what you are doing. And we all have respect for what you did last weekend. I will be honoured if you will accept this.' I finally agree to accept his badge, but there's a pang of guilt that I shouldn't be taking it. A fisherman was killed last week by a vessel that I was captain of, and I just don't think I should receive such a precious gift from these generous people. A few minutes later and Munyos takes me aside, explaining that the badge is a very high honour in the Guatemalan navy, and that he has never heard of anyone giving one away before.

'Capitan. It seems you have friends in high places.' The commandante is standing beside me and I'm sporting a massive hangover, the taste of vodka still in my mouth. I pick up my cell phone and see it's 10am already. 'Last night,' he continues, as I look up at him blearily, 'the President of Guatemala called me. He has issued direct orders that you are to be released, and you can go wherever you like in Guatemala, as long as you are back to meet the judge on Monday. A car will arrive here shortly with two armed guards, and they will take you wherever you would like to go for the weekend. El Presidente also has a beautiful house here in Puerto Quetzal. He says you are his guest now, and you are welcome to stay at his house if you like.'

## As I'm packing my things he sees the gold medal from last night. I'm embarrassed, and not really sure what to say about it

'Thank the President for his generous offer to stay in his house, but I'd really like to go to Antigua to be with my crew please.' As I'm packing my things he sees the gold medal from last night. I'm embarrassed, and not really sure what to say about it. And I'm not sure he'd approve of his men giving away their hard-won medals to people they're supposedly detaining. 'I think,' says the commandante, as I stuff the last of my clothes away, 'that you have many friends who help you.' I look up at him, and he's got that same generous smile. They're a wonderful people here I'm thinking, as El Commandante passes me my crutches.

The arm is raised at the gatehouse and we are waved through. I get my first glimpse of Guatemala outside the military base, and I wonder again at how lucky we are in having so many supporters. Ryan Kiefer, an amazing guy who helped us in Charleston for a couple of weeks, put it very well. '*Earthrace* is like a vortex,' he said. 'There's an energy and magic about *Earthrace* that is very intoxicating. It sucks you in and it's very hard to escape.' This may be close to the truth. The countryside starts to roll by.

Guatemala has had a troubled history, with a recent devastating civil war raging until just 10 years ago, and the country is only now starting to recover. There is an amazing treasure in this country, called Antigua. It is a small city in the mountains about one hour away from Puerto Quetzal. At the start of the war, both sides agreed not to bomb or take refuge in Antigua, realising it was such a key asset for future prosperity, regardless of which side won the war. The hills roll on by and the government car I'm being driven in starts its ascent into the mountains towards Antigua.

In the back seat are two policemen, who speak not a word of English. Driving, though, is Abraham, whose English is outstanding, and he's a wealth of knowledge about this area. We pass an active volcano, a cloud of ash hanging above its peak. 'Beside where you will stay tonight is another active volcano,' he says, 'and if you look at it after dark you will see the red glow from lava.'

The policemen want a photo with me, and we pull over at a lookout and pose, with Abraham taking the shots. An old man comes shuffling by, and his back is laden with firewood, piled so high that he's stooped forwards just to stop from toppling over. He's done it before obviously, because every piece is cut to the same length, and just a single piece of rope binds the whole lot together. Thinking about it, he's probably done this all his life. Down below us I can see hundreds of makeshift houses seemingly randomly cobbled together. Most are just a few sheets of iron strung onto a frame, and many have no separation from one house to the next except for a piece of plywood or a bit of iron. All around this shantytown is a rich array of mountains and lush tropical rainforest, the houses looking like ugly scars on such a wonderful environment.

Two girls come by, probably a similar age to my daughters, and both are carrying large piles of wood on their backs. What a good life my two kids have in comparison, I'm thinking. 'Buenos dias,' I say to them just before they pass. 'Buenos,' they reply in unison, both with big smiles on their faces. The kids go back to talking to each other, blissfully happy, despite the loads on their backs. The people here, I'm learning, are very proud and dignified. There's a certain charm about their immaculate dress sense and the way they conduct themselves. Many of the women wear traditional clothes, but none of the men. 'During the war,' Abraham explains, 'indigenous men were hunted down and shot, or placed into armies, and it was their traditional clothes that sometimes gave them away. So all the men stopped wearing them.' The traditional clothes have patterns and designs from their village, and so people can recognise where

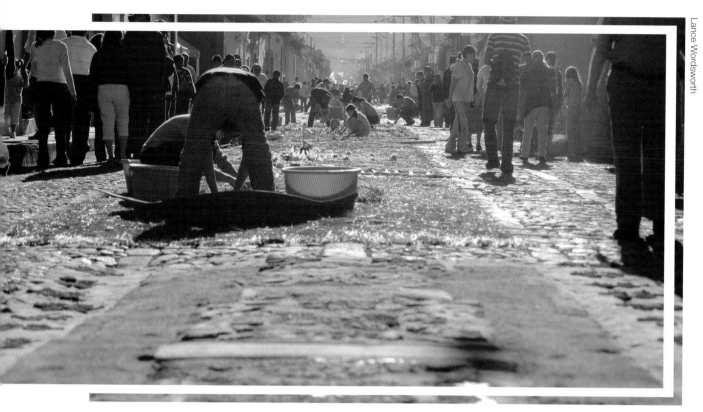

Lance Wordsworth

Families and friends toil all night arranging flowers on the streets that then get trampled by the parade during the day.

you are from simply by your clothes. 'What does this mean?' I say to Abraham, pointing at my worn old Waikato rugby jersey. 'That,' he says with a chuckle, 'means you are a gringo, you are poor, and you will never be married.'

There are a couple of other things I'm learning about the people here. Firstly, they are incredibly happy. It doesn't matter who you meet or what they are doing, they will always have a smile on their face. Secondly, they are extremely courteous. While at the navy base I was always impressed at how polite everyone was, but I'd assumed it was part of the military discipline. It seems this politeness carries on all over the place.

We continue our slow climb up towards Antigua. I'm thinking about these people and the situation they're in. It seems in life we all get dealt a certain set of cards. Some of us get four aces, and some of us get a pair of twos. And what we're all doing in life is just trying to make the most with the hand we've been dealt. I glance at a couple of kids kicking a soccer ball

Lance Wordsworth

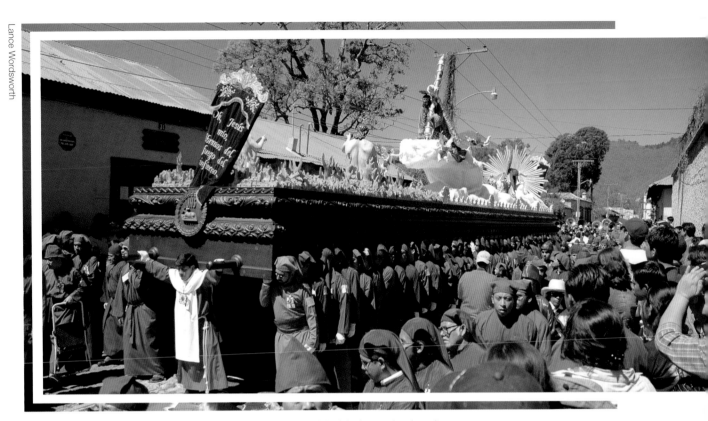

A colourful float goes by in Antigua. This is a wonderful old city tucked up in the mountains in Guatemala.

around on a dirt square. My window is down and I can hear them yelling... but maybe, I wonder, the actual hand you get doesn't matter so much.

We start idling into Antigua, people staring at us curiously. There are wonderful old buildings, many of them hundreds of years old, painted in a myriad of colours. 'There's a big Catholic festival here this weekend,' says Abraham, 'and town will be very busy.' Already there are hundreds of people lining the streets, and our progress drops to a crawl as we navigate to the hotel. Many roads are blocked off, covered for the weekend with stunning artwork and flowerbeds. 'Man, this place is unbelievable,' says Lance as I sling my bag onto the only spare bed left in our tiny hotel room. Ryan comes rolling in, three inches of butt crack showing above his holey underpants. Compared to the locals we must look like a bunch of vagrants. 'This,' says Ryan, 'is one of the coolest places I've ever been.' All the team have a smile on their face. You know, Guatemala ain't so bad.

Five o'clock in the morning, and I'm woken by a few local roosters crowing in the distance. Several hours pass before I extricate myself from my scratcher and hop outside. It's nice and cool up here in the mountains, maybe 15°C. The sky is a deep blue and there's a billow of smoke coming out of the local volcano. I catch a glimpse of Lance filming an old couple as they walk along the cobbled street. The man is laughing at something, and all I can see in his mouth is a single jagged tooth jutting out from his lower jaw. As they come up to the next bed of flowers, they stop and admire it for a few moments, then work their way on down the bustling street.

We wander around town, admiring what must be one of the most amazing mountain cities in the world. Thank goodness our experience of Guatemala didn't end up just being Puerto Quetzal. The food is cheap and amazing. The buildings are ancient and beautiful, and the people are an interesting array of Mayan, Spanish and various other ethnicities that have become part of this landscape.

At three in the afternoon we finally get to see the parade. There are quite literally thousands of men dressed in purple cloaks and pointy hats. Then comes a massive religious float being carried by about 60 men, struggling under its weight. They pant and wheeze as they make their painful journey past us, trampling over the flowers and artwork worshippers had toiled at all night in preparing. It's a loose kind of affair with no police, and people of all persuasions just joining in the procession where they like.

We leave Antigua at about 8am the following day and drive back down the hills to Puerto Quetzal. It's like leaving a sanctuary. This has been such a wonderful stop and we're all disappointed to go, but we have a big day ahead of us.

It's mid morning as we wander into the crowded fast-food restaurant to meet with the fishermen and their families. I start to speak to the group and there's already a sore ache in my throat. Thirty seconds later and I start to cry, and that just sets off a chain reaction among almost everyone there. Ryan across from me is struggling, and he's got tears rolling down his left cheek. Most of the family members are struggling to contain themselves, as I explain how dreadfully sorry my crew and I are with what has happened, and that we know what a tragic loss it has been for them. In my mind I had ideas of remaining composed, but in the end I just lose it. Patrons in the restaurant by now are all staring at us, no doubt wondering what is going on.

Eventually, we settle down, and the group start asking questions through our interpreter. 'When my husband cried out, why did you not rescue him?' This is the poor lady widowed by the accident. I explain that Gonzales was struggling under the skiff, and that because he was closer, I helped him first. By the time I'd swum over to where her husband was he was gone. It's a thought I've had many times since the accident. If I'd swum over to the third fisherman first, I'm sure I'd have rescued him. And my crew would have rescued Gonzalez because he was visible right behind us. But I didn't. I just made my decision at the time and, in hindsight, it was the wrong one.

'Would you mind if we put your husband's name on *Earthrace* as a small tribute to him?' I ask the widow. There's a hush among the group, and they all look at her. She's been crying like many of us and her eyes are red, but now fresh tears start rolling down her cheeks. 'I would be honoured if you would do that for us,' she says through the interpreter. The daughter shows us a photo of her father, and asks that we put 'Pajarito', his nickname, on the boat.

# He has a way of waving his hand in my direction like I'm a grubby little mess to be dealt with

It's an emotional farewell as we get up to leave, but there's a certain satisfaction in having finally met the families and discussed things with them. 'That was one of the hardest things I've ever done,' Ryan says to me, as we're making our way to the courthouse. His eyes are still red and he looks exhausted. 'Yeah, but what wonderful people, eh.' Ryan nods his head, deep in thought. We head up into the courthouse and take our seats.

'Banana banana banana, we wish that Captain Bethune be charged with negligence and imprudence that led to an accident, banana banana banana, that his boat continue to be impounded by the Guatemalan navy, banana banana banana, and that Captain Bethune be detained pending a full court hearing. It is hard to follow every word. I've got English in one ear from Mariana, my interpreter, and Spanish from the public prosecutor in the other.

He's an intimidating-looking man, the prosecutor. He doesn't look at

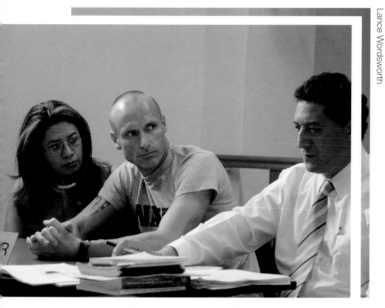

In court with my translator (left) and lawyer (right). Although the proceedings were translated for me, I kept missing things contained within legal jargon.

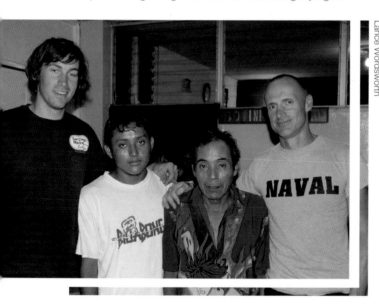

Left to right: Ryan, Carlos Contreras Cruz, Pedro Salazar Gonzalez and myself. It was an emotional roller-coaster meeting with these two and various family members.

me while he's talking, only at the judge, but he has a way of waving his hand in my direction like I'm a grubby little mess to be dealt with. My lawyer stands and presents on my behalf. There is much referring to statutes and existing laws, and eventually I get lost in the translation of legal jargon. He's on my team, though, and it sounds like he's doing a good job.

My one obstacle to freedom remains the prosecutor, who must convince the judge that I should stand trial. I know that under maritime law the case should be clear-cut. The fishing boat was in international waters, it had no solid white light and the crew were asleep, which should see the decision go our way. There are lingering doubts in my mind, though.

I look over to the louvre windows beside the judge, and there's half a dozen small video cameras looking in at me. On the end is one single large lens from our Panasonic HD camera, seemingly out of place among all the handicams. Nice to see Ryan snuck it in. Marian, one of our lawyers, made it abundantly clear no video cameras would be allowed in court, but it seems no one really minds. Suddenly there's a vibration in my pocket, and my phone starts singing a little tune. She'd warned me about this too. 'Turn your cell phones off,' she'd said half an hour earlier. What a nightmare. I've set it up to just keep ringing, and I know it'll just keep singing this little ditty for ages. The judge is looking around for the culprit. I finally manage to extricate it from my pocket. For a fleeting second I think of putting it to my ear and saying something like 'I'd like two fish, three hot dogs and five dollars' chips thanks'. Common sense prevails and I turn it off. The judge is clearly not

impressed, and the court remains quiet as she sits there glaring at me, no one saying a word. My lawyer has his head in his hands. 'Umm. Sorry about that,' I mumble at my interpreter.

Eventually, the judge starts announcing her decision. It takes her ages to get to the point. But then it comes. 'The collision was an accident, and was not caused by negligence or imprudence on the part of Captain Bethune. He is free to leave Guatemala when he likes. And he is free to take his boat whenever and wherever he likes.' That was the translation at least. And I will remember those words for the rest of my life. Freedom — here we come.

Later in the day we pay a visit to Gonzalez, who is still recovering in hospital. His family from the meeting earlier in the day are there already, and they greet us like friends as we walk in. He's a tiny little man, but there's a certain wiry strength about him. I remember lifting him onto the stretcher and being amazed at how heavy he was. We go through a question-and-answer session with him. It turns out he actually went under the main hull of *Earthrace* as we rode over the skiff.

# Two big curved scars, one across each shoulder blade and, by the look of them, probably matching our propeller blades

He takes his shirt off to reveal a massive scar from his sternum all the way down his belly. He seems quite proud of it really. His belly was cut open by surgeons to repair his stomach, intestine and fractured sternum. Then Ryan sees the scars on his back. 'Hey, check these out Pete.' We never saw these cuts on the night. Two big curved scars, one across each shoulder blade and, by the look of them, probably matching our propeller blades. We're lucky he's alive I reckon.

It's been an emotional roller-coaster of a day, but one that we'll never forget. The families were left in no doubt that we were sorrowful for what had happened, and that we did our very best on the night to rescue the fishermen. The accident has forever changed their lives, however, and all the crew realise there is nothing we can do to bring the dead fisherman back. Hopefully, the insurance money and meeting us here today will help

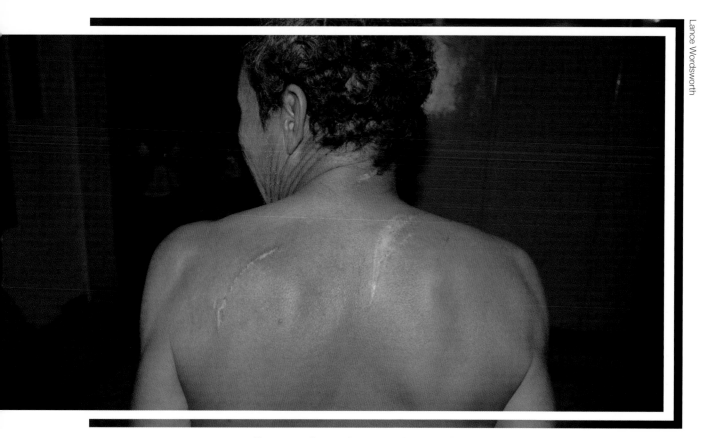

Lance Wordsworth

Two propeller marks on the back of Gonzalez. He was quite proud of his scars.

in some way to them moving on. These people are desperately poor by our standards, but there's also a great sense of community and family spirit among them, and I'm hopeful they'll be OK.

We say our goodbyes to the navy people, undock and silently head out of the harbour. Something, though, is not quite right with the port gearbox. As soon as we load up the engines, it slips. There's a sudden grinding, and I'm thinking the gearbox is stuffed, maybe from damage caused in the collision. 'Actually,' says Scott, 'when you're in the engine room, it is more like popping noises from fluid.' Which of course doesn't sound good, but it's probably better than grinding gears.

Scott sits reading the ZF manual. 'We should try bypassing the solenoid and force it into forward manually,' he says after some time, and he disappears into the engine room. A few minutes later and there's a sudden lurch forward as the manual override kicks in, but no sign of any slippage. I look down at the loads, and both port and starboard are reading the same. A few more revs and it seems like forward has been engaged properly on the port gearbox. Scott emerges looking pleased.

'Just don't put it into reverse or the whole thing will explode to bits,' he says.

We're not entirely sure what is wrong with the gearbox — perhaps a damaged clutch or faulty solenoid. Either way, it'll be easier to get it sorted in Acapulco, or better still San Diego if it makes it that far.

Right now we're in forward, and we'll leave it there till we're well into Mexican waters. 'We're on our way,' I call to Ryan and Lance, who are busy editing software for one of the TV networks. They look up at me, smiling, but not overjoyed. Guatemala has cast a long shadow over *Earthrace*, and while we're pleased to be leaving, there's certainly no elation in it. We're just grateful to be on our way again.

The gearbox holds all the way to Mexico, and we dock in the resort town of Acapulco. It's an intimidating line of biodiesel drums that awaits us as we start the refuelling operation. One 12-volt pump and two little petrol pumps hum away as the barrels are gradually emptied. Four hours later and we're off, on our way to San Diego in California.

We're only an hour into the next leg before we hit trouble. The whistle from the starboard engine turbo starts to change, its tone moving up and down, as the engine starves for fuel. Scampering into the engine room, I see the Racor filter system is showing high vacuum, indicating a blocked filter. Switching the Racor filter over to a new cartridge, the vacuum drops away and the engine returns to its normal drone.

'What was it?' says Allison, as I emerge into the galley.

'This,' and I scrape my finger along the filter, removing a thin layer of brown, grease-like stuff caked along the filter sides. 'It's glycerine. The fuel we picked up in Acapulco must be dodgy.'

Allison looks at my finger and scowls. 'What can we do about it?'

'We'll just have to keep changing filters every time they block, and hope we have enough of them to get to San Diego.' She shakes her head at me, and wanders back into the helm muttering.

I follow her through, picking up the logbook to write down the event. I've just finished when the little green light on our dashboard comes on. I like this light. It tells me there's an email waiting.

'Who is it?' asks Allison.

'It's from Scott. He reckons we should have flat seas all the way, which is hard to believe when we've got snotty weather already.' I look out the port window, and there's solid two-metre waves coming at us.

'Let's just hope it is a small system which clears.'

Six hours later and the waves have gradually built to an awkward three metres. It is funny how waves are different all over the world. These ones here are what I'd call consistent. They are packed closely together in gangs, not threatening us in any way, but big enough to cause discomfort. The only nice thing about them is they are regular in direction and pitch. There remain serious vibrations coming through the drive-train as a result of collision damage, so we've limited our speed to around 15 knots. As a result we're only partially piercing the waves, which makes for an awkward ride.

'I've had enough of this,' says Ryan finally. He's in the navigator's chair trying to eat some chicken soup.

## 'There's water leaking in here from somewhere'

'It's why they call this the Baja bash,' Allison explains. 'The weather is nearly always crap heading up to the Baja Peninsula.' There's a whoosh as we pierce a wave, and Ryan swears as a big dollop of soup lands in his lap.

'There's water leaking in here from somewhere,' says Allison. On the floor right by the helm is a telltale puddle of water, leaking in from somewhere. But finding the leak is not so easy. It is working its way down a labyrinth of carbon structures. We eventually track it to a small hole in the roof where the new sat phone antenna goes through. I look up in the hole and see there's no silicone in there to seal it. 'Who was the dodgy engineer who did that?' I wonder out loud. There's no point trying to fix it while water continues to come through, so we decide to sort it in San Diego when we can dry it out properly. In the meantime the water continues its evil little journey down beside the helm, mocking us.

The bashing continues unabated for three days, as do multiple filter changes. None of us sleeps well, and we're all now showing the effects. Scott's forecasts keep telling us the weather is about to improve, but it keeps getting worse. 'You know the worst thing about the weather,' says Ryan, 'is that everything becomes such a chore. Brushing your teeth, cooking, cleaning, changing, sleeping, it all gets so damned difficult when it's rough.'

I look down at the FLIR infra-red night vision system. A much bigger wave comes racing towards us, and I can see it in a strange grey-scale image as it rears over the helm. It is like watching some kind of PlayStation game, only in this case the result is real, as a sudden wave of energy envelops us. *Earthrace* punches out the back of the wave and hits an enormous trough in a bone-jarring crash. 'Can this boat handle such abuse?' says Allison, with a look of concern on her face.

'Well,' I respond, 'the designers reckon the limiting factor is the violence the crew will tolerate rather than what the boat can handle.'

'Which means what?' she asks. I think about this a minute. *Earthrace* is certainly one of the toughest race boats ever built. It has been through two different storms with 12-metre waves that terrified the crew, but came out unscathed. These waves here are only around four metres. What worries me, though, is the repetitiveness of the impacts. It's been almost non-stop for three days now, and I'm worried we'll get a stress fracture or two sneaking into the structure.

'Well, I think we'll be fine,' I say to Allison finally, trying to sound confident.

I wander down to the toilet, sit on the seat, and brace myself against the wall. This is a tricky operation when it's rough like this, and I've been putting it off, hoping the conditions would improve with the change in tide — which they haven't. It's not a successful operation either.

'The toilet is all blocked,' I say to Ryan. He looks at me and shakes his head. I've always given him a hard time for blocking it, and to be fair he normally has been the culprit.

'I'm going to hold on till San Diego,' he says determinedly. 'We should be there by lunchtime.'

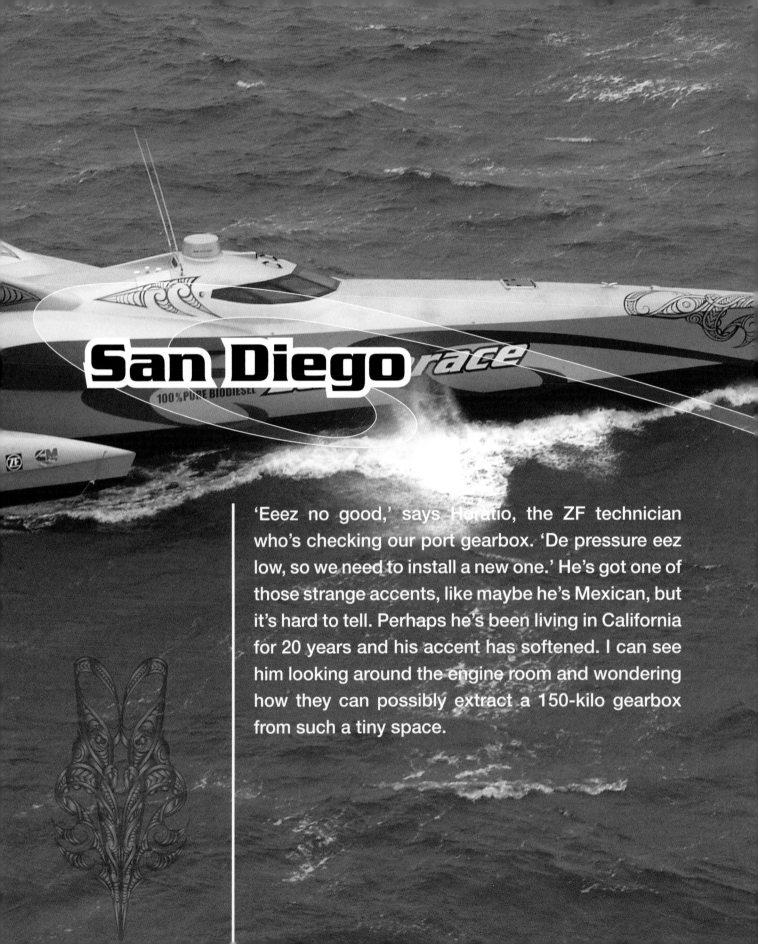

# San Diego

'Eeez no good,' says Horatio, the ZF technician who's checking our port gearbox. 'De pressure eez low, so we need to install a new one.' He's got one of those strange accents, like maybe he's Mexican, but it's hard to tell. Perhaps he's been living in California for 20 years and his accent has softened. I can see him looking around the engine room and wondering how they can possibly extract a 150-kilo gearbox from such a tiny space.

Scott looks up from behind the gearbox. 'I reckon the clutch plates were smashed in the collision in Guatemala. It's the only way to explain the loss in gear pressure.' Horatio nods in agreement. He's still frowning, though, now looking at our tiny doorway.

'I don't sink we can fit da gearbox out.'

'Oh, don't worry,' says Scott. 'We'll sort something.'

I head down to the sleeping quarters to get some shut-eye. Replacing a gearbox is a massive job, and there are plenty of people here to help. The last few days catch up on me, and in a matter of minutes I'm asleep.

I'm woken by a strange sawing noise. I can hear the lads chatting away down in the engine room, and Anthony (who is back helping us out in San Diego) is busy with a hacksaw, cutting out a square section of wall to fit the gearbox out. 'Man, Pete will be pissed when he sees this,' he says, laughing, as he pulls out a large section of sandwich composite. I watch them from the dark sleeping quarters, feeling a bit like a peeping Tom. I don't mind them cutting the wall out at all. You gotta do what you gotta do, and right now we need the damaged gearbox out and the new one in. I drift back to sleep with the guys grunting away in the background as the massive gearbox is handled into the cockpit.

## What an amazing effort. To change a gearbox overnight like that is impressive indeed

It's 6am before I wake up and wander outside. Horatio and Scott are there, both looking exhausted. Horatio's eyes are bloodshot, like he's been drinking all night. 'How'd ya get on?' I ask.

'Eeez all done,' he says, with a nonplussed look on his face. 'I'm going home now to sleep.' What an amazing effort. To change a gearbox overnight like that is impressive indeed. Horatio, though, is typical of the ZF technicians. Of all the companies we've worked with, ZF have impressed me the most. Their engineers are all outstanding, both technically and in their work ethic.

The crew finish loading up and we head out for a sea trial, conscious of not losing any more time. Ryan and I have got big smiles on our faces. We got off lightly here. Only a half day lost and we've now got a new gearbox. Our elation is short-lived, however, as Marty, our new engineer, comes running into the helm. 'Hey Pete, you'd better take a look at this.' We clamber

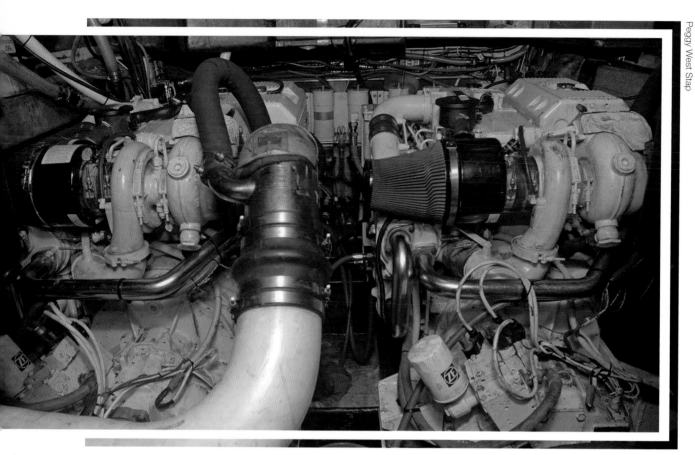

Peggy West Stap

Two Cummins Mercruiser Diesel QSC-540 engines. A lot of grunt from relatively small engines. Behind the engines are ZF-305A gearboxes.

into the engine room, and Marty points to the starboard driveshaft, now wobbling all over the place. We turn around and head back into Shelter Island in San Diego, not knowing exactly what is wrong, but conscious we need to sort it.

It's late in the afternoon before Scott emerges with a verdict. 'One of the engine mounts has collapsed, so we're not going anywhere until we get a new one.' He and Allison order one from Maine, while the rest of us head back to the hotel, resigned to the fact that we're here for at least another day.

I'm busy sorting my washing when Lance comes running out of the bathroom. 'Hey, look what I've caught,' and he proffers his hand towards us with a single square of toilet paper on it. We all look at the hostile centipede crawling around on the paper. It takes a few shuffles forward, digs its pincers into the paper, and shakes its head angrily as it tries to burrow in. It gives up and moves forward a few more paces before trying again.

'And why exactly are you showing us this?' asks Allison, somewhat perplexed at Lance's excitement. He explains he's been seeing these in his poos for a week or so now, and he's only just managed to catch one. He has the proud look of a fisherman who's finally caught a 20-pound snapper. 'The plan from here,' he continues, 'is to get one of the local doctors to look at it, and then get a treatment.' By now the little sucker has managed to get a bit of a hole started in the toilet paper, no doubt hoping it can burrow all the way back into Lance's warm and snuggly bottom.

Scott returns and we head out to dinner. It's actually my birthday, and given there's not much we can do until the mount arrives we may as well enjoy ourselves. 'Here ya go,' says John, handing me a rum and coke. This is the first bit of alcohol I've had in ages. I put the glass to my lips. It tastes sweet and delicious, and the familiar smell of it is comforting, like an old friend. By the time the second one is finished my head is already blurry. What a cheap date I am these days!

John comes back over, not with a drink this time but his mobile. 'It's one of your girls.'

'Hey, Dad, happy birthday.' It's Danielle, and she's got the voice normally reserved for when she wants something. 'Can you catch me another possum, because I really miss Blossom?' Blossom was a pet possum we'd had a year or so ago. My mind wanders back to the cheeky little blighter scrambling up my leg . . . and Danielle biking up the road with the possum sitting on her head, its tail curled back around her neck. It was actually quite a cool pet.

'Yeah, I might be able to get you another Blossom,' I say, suddenly missing Sharyn and my girls.

It's a strange journey — all this time away from our families, and for what? We've just pounded ourselves senseless for days crossing the Baja, in the hope of still getting a record, and yet here we are stuck in San Diego, making the record even tougher to get. It feels like we're digging a hole, and all we seem to be doing is making the hole deeper. And yet there is still a quiet optimism among the team that we will do it, despite the ever-mounting odds stacked against us. Scott had said the other day that this is all happening for a reason, we just don't know what that reason is yet. Maybe it's so we have such enormous odds to overcome, and we'll then sneak the record by one hour in Barbados, which will make for an unbelievable TV series. Or maybe it's to pummel us into submission and we'll crawl back to New Zealand with our tails between our legs.

An email came through today from a young girl in New York. 'What you do matters,' she said. 'What you have achieved already is special, but please don't give up, because we all believe in you.' It is a humbling experience to get emails like this from people you've never met, offering support. I guess the crew all believe what we're doing does matter or we wouldn't be putting ourselves through all this.

The following day we're down at the boatyard nice and early. I look over on the dock beside us and there's a face that seems vaguely familiar. He's pulling lines on this old-looking yacht and it hits me: Dennis Connor, of America's Cup fame. Well, we're docked in prestigious company indeed. He won the cup in Fremantle and also lost it here in San Diego. He looks like he's been eating pretty well since then, and his face is weathered like you'd expect on an old sea dog. 'How's it going Dennis?' I say, as I wander up beside him like he's an old friend. A frown crosses his face and then he grimaces.

## He needs to get his boat to New York, and I need to get mine around the world

'Well,' he says, 'the cranes stuffed things yesterday, they've stuffed things again today, nothing is going right, and I'm supposed to have this boat in New York next week.' He looks down at his boat, *Stars n Stripes*, then wanders off without looking back. He has a lot on his mind, I guess. In fact, we all do. He needs to get his boat to New York, and I need to get mine around the world.

Allison comes scuttling down the dock with a very stressed look on her face. 'The mounts are still stuck in Maine,' she blurts out. 'The tosser never sent them at all.' Oh man. Stink one. His excuse is that DHL won't accept the shipment because he isn't registered. Something to do with 9/11 he says. Yeah right. They're just a bit of metal and rubber.

Half an hour later and Allison has more news. 'There are four mounts in Texas that will fit, but we can't have them until 8am tomorrow morning.' I wonder if they really will arrive. We're rapidly losing faith in US courier companies and promises of delivery. 'Make sure you get tracking numbers and we keep tabs on where these things are,' I growl at her unfairly.

The engine mounts do in fact arrive the following day, and Scott is quick to get them installed. This improves the situation somewhat, but doesn't fix it entirely. 'It's like there are multiple things causing vibrations. The engine mount was just one of them,' says Scott. We debate what else could be causing the problems. A bad injector in the engine would certainly cause vibrations, the driveshaft could be bent, or the coupling could be damaged. Or even a combination of these. The propeller could be out, although they were replaced with new ones in Guatemala so they should be fine.

'Let's just start working through them, starting with the injectors,' I say, and Scott disappears to call the Cummins Mercruiser guys.

Lance comes back along the dock. 'How goes the worm?' asks Allison.

'Well, I went and saw a doctor this morning and he has no idea what it is. He's given me a worm treatment in case, but reckons it might not work because what I have are actually centipedes.'

'Why don't we just post an image of it on the website and see if any kids can recognise it? Maybe make it a competition where they win some *Earthrace* goodies.'

Lance looks over at Allison and frowns. 'Oh, that's just brilliant. Tell the whole world about the animals living up my bum. I'll never get a girlfriend again.'

'Yeah, but should you even have a girlfriend with those things crawling around? At least this way you might be able to get it sorted.' Lance finally agrees, and wanders off to load the images onto our website.

The Cummins Mercruiser technicians arrive, and determine quickly that one injector is indeed bad. They replace it, and then during sea trials we find that the low-speed vibration has now gone but high-speed vibrations remain. 'Well, we're still making improvements,' says Scott. 'But it ain't fixed, which means we need to pull the prop and driveshaft.' Marty has a horrified look on his face.

'There is no way you can pull the shaft without pulling *Earthrace* from the water.' He looks to the others for support, but most of the team are not really sure. Except for Scott.

'Sure it can. Just get a few ropes and it'll come out no worries.'

Marty shakes his head in disbelief. 'And how are you getting the shaft back in?' he enquires.

'We'll just do the reverse,' say Scott enthusiastically. 'Come on, man. This is *Earthrace*.'

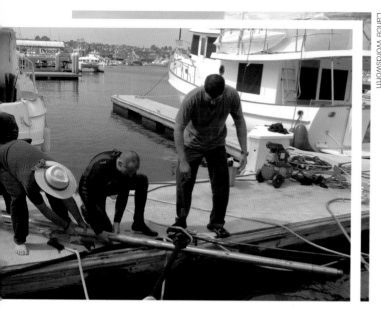

Left to right: Ryan, Scott, me and Marty Mead after we'd removed the three-inch propeller shaft from *Earthrace*.

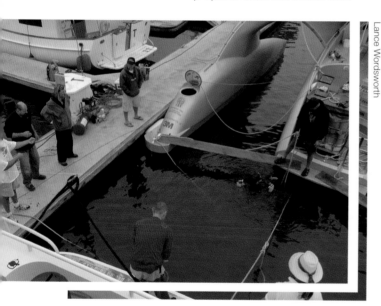

It was a real mission installing the propeller shaft. We ended up with a spider's web of ropes. Here it is beneath *Earthrace*, and Ryan is in the water giving us all instructions to line it up and force it through the shaft bearings.

I think back to Charleston where *Earthrace* was out of the water. We pulled the starboard prop shaft out and it was such a mission, let alone doing it under water. I'm starting to wonder if Marty is right. Scott seems confident, though, so I wander forward to get the dive gear ready.

The water looks cold and uninviting. I'm squeezing into my Orca wetsuit and looking at the dark water. California water never gets that warm, apparently. I drop down off the transom step of *Earthrace* into it, and a chill runs through me as the water works its way under the neoprene rubber. 'Harden up, ya wuss,' says Ryan, when he sees I'm not enjoying it. I'm waiting for the hammer gun, and getting colder by the second.

A few minutes later and we're removing the port propeller. We've done it so many times now that it doesn't take long. Next comes the hard part, getting the shaft out. An old sea dog from one of the boats next to us comes wandering past. 'You're doing what?' he says in disbelief, when he hears we're removing the prop shaft. 'You'll sink ya damn boat,' he says as he wanders off, shaking his head.

We rig up ropes and pulleys from a boat astern of us, from the transom step and from the dock, and gradually the shaft starts to budge. Marty, now buried in the engine room, suddenly starts yelling. 'Water is pissing everywhere!' The three-inch section of shaft is past the seal, but the end of the shaft is not, so he's got a gaping wound allowing water in. 'Hurry up guys, this bilge is filling up fast,' he yells, sounding even more desperate. We lean back on the main pull line and suddenly the whole lot comes shooting right out and our 4.5-metre, stainless steel shaft goes plummeting to the sea bed. Marty quickly wedges a wooden plug in the shaft hole, sealing her up, while the rest of us start the laborious task of hauling the shaft up onto the dock. A few minutes later and five of us triumphantly carry the 150-kilogram shaft on our shoulders out to a waiting pickup, much to the amusement of the yard workers.

A couple of hours later and Allison is back with both the propeller and the shaft. 'All sorted,' she says smiling. 'The propeller was five grams out, and the shaft was 17 thou out, and they're all fixed.' Five grams on a propeller probably wouldn't cause much vibration, but 17 thou on the shaft certainly would. I cross my fingers, hoping the problem has been fixed.

The shaft is tied up on the dock and lowered down into the water behind *Earthrace*. 'Now don't cock this up,' says Scott, 'or we'll be here for another week repairing a busted P-bracket.' He and I are both worried about this. Once we get the shaft end into the bracket, it must be held at the right height as it gets fed in. If not it'll be a disaster. There are now eight of us laboriously manoeuvring the shaft into position, with Ryan in the water guiding us. The end goes in, then a couple of inches more. Inch by inch we crank the shaft through the P-bracket and line it up on the second shaft bearing.

'Pull on those lines!' I yell at the guys on the winch.

'The winch handle is about to break,' David complains. 'I can't get any more pressure.'

I look down at the shaft. It's like a giant silver eel sneaking into *Earthrace*. The ropes on the shaft are all tight, trying to push it home, but it just isn't budging. By now a small crowd has gathered around to enjoy the spectacle.

John and I hurry over to the line directly above the shaft end and jiggle it up and down. I can feel the play of the shaft in the bearing. Suddenly it all lines up and the shaft shoots right up through the second shaft bearing. Everyone hauls and it is pushed home. 'Man, how good are we?' says Scott triumphantly. There's high fives all round as we admire our achievement. The old sea dog who'd said we'd sink our boat has been watching from the dock. 'Well, captain,' he says with a slight Dutch accent, 'I am impressed.' He's impressed — man, I'm amazed.

We head out for a sea trial, and the drive-train feels nicely balanced. No hint of vibrations anywhere. 'As smooth as silk,' says Scott with satisfaction, as we turn around and head back to Shelter Island to load up.

# Pacific crossing

It's almost dark by the time we slip out of our dock in San Diego. A US Customs boat passes and gives us a wave. Then a navy patrol vessel sneaks by for a look. It's amazing all this resource employed around the US coastline. This last week we've seen Coastguard, Navy, Customs, Maritime Police, plus some dodgy-looking guys in a camouflaged RIB who were probably Counter-Terrorist Group or special forces. Then there are all the Coastguard and military choppers patrolling up and down the coastline.

'Why do you need so many patrols?' I had asked one of the US Coastguard guys earlier in the week.' He'd been surprised by the question, I guess assuming all countries had lots of military patrolling their waters. 'Because we have a lot of enemies,' he'd replied, after giving it some thought.

A nice rolling Pacific greets us. 'I love this ocean,' I say to Harold, who has joined us for this one leg to Hawaii. He looks bemused, wondering why you'd love one ocean over any other. I'm from the Pacific, albeit some five thousand miles away from where we are now. It is the largest ocean on earth, the deepest, and supports the most fish life. It also has these beautiful rolling swells that go for thousands of miles, making wicked surfing when they finally reach land.

# This is my ocean, I think to myself, as I watch the sun setting on the horizon

I think back to last July when we'd crossed this ocean on our way from New Zealand to Vancouver. It feels like a lifetime ago. We'd caught a big wahoo and a barracuda on the way over. There are still lots of fish left in this ocean, unlike other waters, which are increasingly fished out. This is my ocean, I think to myself, as I watch the sun setting on the horizon in front of me.

The smell of hot butter and eggs wafts down into the sleeping quarters where Ryan is just waking. He stirs and looks up towards the galley where I'm busy cooking breakfast. 'What's cooking bro?' he asks expectantly. Ryan is like a trap-door spider for any cooked food.

'Sausages and eggs,' I reply, knowing he'll turn his nose up at the sausages part. He's a vegetarian of sorts, and because he arranges most of the food for *Earthrace*, for a while now we've been on a semi-vegetarian diet. The trouble is I see no reason to get to the top of the food chain and then just eat fruit and veges — good as those things are. So this morning I'm cooking sausages, although I've struggled to get normal pork sausages like we'd cook on a barbecue back home. Allison has been buying sausage rolls and lots of weird sausage meats for us, despite my pleas for just plain pork sausages.

It's a beautiful morning, and we are between two weather systems. To the north, there is a storm gradually abating, and we can see its telltale clouds in the distance, and to the south is another system, which is gradually growing in strength. Right now we're handily tucked between the two, with beautiful seas and a gentle rolling swell from the north. I wander onto the back deck with my breakfast.

The temperature is starting to warm up. It feels like 25°C already. I whip my shirt off and lie in the sun with my kai sitting in my lap. The sun feels hot, but I know I won't get sunburned here. The ozone is thick, protecting me from the harmful UV rays that wreak havoc down under. In New Zealand, the skin cancer rate is three times that of the US, despite New Zealand also consuming triple the amount of sunscreen per capita. And yet it was Europe and the US that produced most of the ozone-depleting CFCs in the 1970s and '80s. It highlights that our actions may impact on others in unexpected ways, and sometimes this is felt on the opposite side of the globe. It is something I've pondered many times in the last year or so.

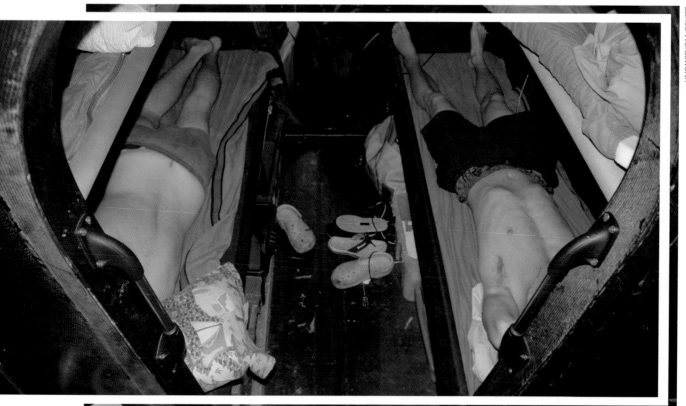

Ryan and me catching up on sleep. Normally Ryan has a lot more crack showing.

Lance Wordsworth

Increasingly, I believe that what each of us does matters, because it affects other people, now and in the future.

I look up at the tattered New Zealand flag flying from our port VHF aerial. Twelve months ago it was brand spanking; now it's a tattered mess only half the length of what it was. The section with four stars is all but weathered away, and it could just as easily pass for an Australian flag now. 'We should get someone to send us a new one,' says Ryan, who sometimes seems like he's reading my mind. I ponder this for a moment. There's a charm about the bedraggled flag hanging there. It's been on *Earthrace* from day one, and has faithfully weathered all the storms and harsh conditions we've put it through. 'You know Ryan, I kinda like the old flag. I reckon we'll leave it mate.' There's a new US flag ready to go on the starboard aerial, probably twice the size of the humble old Kiwi flag.

# Day 31 and we're over 4000 nautical miles behind the time we have to beat

'Pete, do you really think we have any chance of getting the record now?' Ryan asks earnestly. It's a tough question. We lost three days in Panama, 11 days in Guatemala after the collision, and another six days in San Diego repairing the damage. So all up we've already lost 20 days. We're now on day 31 and we're over 4000 nautical miles behind the time we have to beat. I went through the numbers last night, and if we had an amazing run with basically no lost time from here, we could still get the record. What are the odds, I wonder? 'Well,' I reply, 'we're still in with a chance mate, but we need a great run from here.' Ryan throws me a dubious glance then goes back to admiring our flag. I'm not sure if he believes me or not. But all we can do is our best, as we always have. And if that is good enough, fantastic. If it isn't, at least we tried.

There's my star. I've seen it the last three nights on my shift from 2 to 4am. It's brighter than those around it; perhaps it's not too far from earth. My friendly star keeps going in and out of view behind the massive carbon mullions that support the windscreen. It's an unusual windscreen on *Earthrace*: more like a race car than a boat. It is small, wrapping around you, only offering small sections to see through, but it's also like a small cocoon keeping us safe from the destructive seas just a few metres away.

The windscreen is designed to go down to seven metres under water, with a factor of safety of three. 'So at 21 metres under water it all implodes on you,' Craig Loomes had said to me with a glint in his eye at one of our meetings. In sea trials around New Zealand we experienced five metres of wave on top of the windscreen, as we went through some enormous 12-metre waves. It was one of the scariest experiences of my life, and something I never want to repeat. So bugger seven metres under water, I think to myself, let alone 21 metres.

It's now 2.30am and everyone else is asleep. Time for the few jobs I have at night. I scurry down to the engine bay and check the bank of Racor filters. All close to zero. Sweet. Next I check the fuel levels in our main and day tanks. We're slightly down on fuel, which surprises me. Not sure why, but I'll figure it out in the morning I tell myself, as I pop back into the driver's seat. I look out to starboard and my star is still there, waiting for me.

The waves feel a little different now, certainly bigger than before, but also slightly more from starboard. I switch my radar over to the FLIR night vision system to take a look. They've grown to about three metres in height, and are just verging on where we'll be able to surf them. A wave comes through and picks up our stern, pointing our bow down into the trough in front. The turbocharger whistle drops slightly, and we're carried along for a short time, before dropping off the back of the wave. Not quite surfing yet, but if these waves build any more it'll be a great surf all the way to Hawaii.

Three o'clock ticks over on the engine control panel — time for a feed. I fossick around in our small refrigerator. There tucked at the bottom under a manky old lettuce is a boysenberry yoghurt — you little beauty! Amazing that this slipped past Ryan, who's normally first to finish all the good stuff. A quick look in the galley for an orange. Just three left. Well, it's now two, as I grab one of them and wander back to the helm. Food fills a big part of our day, and I use it as a way to break up my shifts at night.

I plug my iPod in and put it on shuffle. I'd probably be mad without this, I think to myself. 'Well, who says you're not mad already?' says the second voice that keeps talking to me. When I look back over the last 12 months of adventures, I associate different periods with certain bands. On the New Zealand tour, it was Kora. For the Pacific crossing it was The Postal Service and for the US tour it was the new Conscious Roots album. I'm not sure what it'll be for the race yet. I haven't had much time to get new music loaded.

I glance down at the engine controls: 3.57am. Time to wake Ryan for his shift. I wander down to the sleeping quarters, and he's lying on his side with his mouth open. His face is glowing from the red Hella LED lights. There's a good reason why we use these. Under red light, the human eye maintains a dilated pupil, helping with night vision. When exposed to white light, however, the pupil will partially close, reducing vision in low light. Not that Ryan cares about red lights right now. I rock his shoulder for a few seconds until he stirs. I don't need to say anything. He just looks at me disappointedly, and starts his ritual of waking himself up, which normally takes about three minutes. Ahh, my scratcher looks inviting.

It's early the following morning when a sudden shudder starts driving through *Earthrace*. The entire hull shakes violently and there's a thumping noise coming from the aft somewhere. My heart sinks as I imagine our port drive-train broken and in tatters.

# The entire hull shakes violently and there's a thumping noise coming from the aft somewhere

We disengage the gears and run outside. Emerging from under the transom step is an evil-looking mess of nets and ropes. 'Just some old fishing gear stuck in the prop,' says Marty nonchalantly. I grab a dive mask and spit in it to stop it fogging, then rinse it in salt water. In I go to survey the damage, which to my surprise is not that bad. Just a tight ball of rope wrapped around the propeller shaft, and a big tail of nets that Marty is busy pulling on. The propeller blades all look fine, and no damage to the hull. I grab a serrated knife and hack the main rope away from the shaft, and Marty pulls the rest of it aboard.

The water here is over five miles deep and has a beautiful deep blue colour. It is also amazingly clear. I take a quick look around to make sure there are no sharks lurking. Not that there would be in a remote spot like this, but I look nonetheless. I then dive down about five metres and look up at the hull. I can see all the way to the bow, some 24 odd metres away. I like the Pacific, I remind myself again.

Back on *Earthrace* the cluster of ropes and net lie like a carcass on the deck. It's made up of many different ropes and nets, all bound together in a tangled mess. 'Been around for ages,' says Marty, pointing at the algal growth. It has probably been out here for years, drifting at the whim of Pacific currents.

Marty puts *Earthrace* back in gear and we get under way again towards Hawaii. I'm still not sure about Marty. Technically I think he's pretty good, but he's also used to being captain of his own boat, rather than an engineer under someone else. Not easy, though, fitting in with an existing crew that's been together for ages. And it's early days.

Two days later we approach Maui. Ryan suddenly jumps from his seat, yelling he's seen a whale right in front of us. A few seconds later and an enormous humpback whale breaches the surface, coming right out of the water, and then crashing down into a spray of white water and froth.

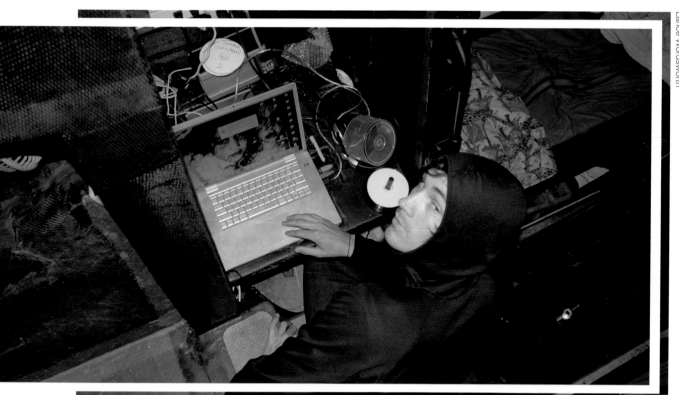

Ryan built this little desk to edit video footage during the race. It sits between the helm and the sleeping quarters.

Lance Wordsworth

Seconds later, another smaller whale does the same. Then a third one careers out of the blue water directly in front of us. Apparently, there's not that much food here for whales. They just come to show off and breed.

Half an hour later and we're pulling into Maalaia on Maui. 'Oh wicked, check that out,' Ryan says as we enter the harbour. There at the entrance is a lone Maori kuia or old woman intoning a karanga or call; it is a traditional greeting by hosts that acknowledges the visitors and pays tribute to the departed. There's something very spiritual about this person as her call carries out over the harbour towards us, rather mournful, almost sad, welcoming us in. For a few seconds I'm lost in memories of back home. 'Man, are we privileged,' Ryan says as we pass her.

As we drift up to the dock, a group of six Maori warriors begin a haka. 'Ka mate, ka mate' resounds around the harbour, and the local journalists and film crews all turn to the group of Maori. We are blessed indeed.

Our jobs during refuelling are pretty much delegated already. We all scurry off to work on them, while I hang around to meet with media. 'Do you still have any chance of getting the record?' is their first question. I dutifully explain that, yes, we do still have a chance, but it is a very big challenge from here. Among the media people is a German film crew who'd flown over specially to meet us.

A few hours later and we're packed and back out to sea, on our way to the Marshall Islands. 'You know,' says Ryan, hacking into a big bowl of Thai green curry, 'that would be one of the coolest stops we've ever had.' It was special: there were the whales, the karanga and haka to welcome us, all the locals there to wish us well, a good media turnout, a blessing of the boat. I have to admit it was awesome.

'I mean,' continues Ryan, 'what about that chick Tina preparing all this grub for us?' I look down at my bowl of curry, which surprisingly I've finished ahead of Ryan. I have to admit it is amazing. We'd met Tina on our brief stopover in Maui last year, and she'd promised to help with food when we came back . . . and help she did. What she's prepared is five days' worth of precooked meals, with the ingredients and sauces all listed as to what goes with what. And the food is outstanding. We've polished off the green curry, and for dinner tomorrow it's going to be prawns with black bean Thai sauce.

'Why is it that people are so helpful to us?' Ryan adds. It's a good question, and one that we've thought about many times.

'Some support us because we're promoting biodiesel. Some like our attitudes towards the environment in general. Some probably like to be part of this amazing adventure. And a few probably feel sorry for all the tough times we're enduring.' Although not so tough today, I reflect, as Ryan stuffs a final spoonful of curry into his wide-open mouth.

'Yeah, but we only met her for a couple of hours. I still can't see why she's done all this,' Ryan says, pointing at the mountain of prepacked food. He can be like a dog with a bone on things sometimes.

While in Maui a film crew had said to me, 'What do you want to achieve out of Earthrace?' and at the time I didn't answer it that eloquently. But on reflection later, Earthrace is about connecting with people. Some we connect with only marginally. Maybe they've read a newspaper article on *Earthrace* or seen the boat in a harbour. But some we definitely connect with more strongly and they tend to be the ones who get to go aboard *Earthrace* or meet us in person. I go on to explain to Ryan that Tina must be one of them. He looks almost satisfied with the answer, as he wipes the sauce off his chin, having finally chewed his way through the last mouthful. He pats his stomach and has a satisfied grin.

'Well, whatever the reason, it sure is good to have her on our side.'

The following day and our toilet is blocked again. Since launching, the toilet has been our most unreliable piece of equipment. Much of the problem, though, has been the other bits connected to the toilet that are part of the overall system, such as the wiring, holding tank and saltwater pump. In the last 12 months I reckon we've only had about two months with a working bog. Generally, what we've done is stop, hang our bum over the transom step, and let it go. And every now and then you'll get a wave shooting up ya bum like an oversized saltwater bidet. Today, however, we're in race mode, and stopping isn't an option.

I look back through the galley and there is Ryan, staring in disgust at the toilet, the contents of which have turned into an ugly, brown, lumpy soup, sloshing around in the bowl. 'Don't worry mate, just use that,' I say, pointing at the bright new orange bucket we'd picked up in Hawaii. Ryan throws me a dirty look and wanders back to the sleeping quarters, no doubt deciding to clench his cheeks for a while. Using a bucket sure isn't appealing, but neither is pulling the toilet to bits and repairing it. I'd fixed the toilet once last year and it was the most disgusting job I've ever done.

Marty comes creeping out of the sleeping quarters, still half asleep, and with his eyes half closed. 'Hey, can ya fix the toilet mate? Must be blocked or something,' I say to him, as nonchalantly as I can.

'Sure thing,' he replies, as he throws a couple of slices of bread in the toaster.

I look out the side window and there is a plover flying along next to us, every now and then dipping down to skim the water, then rising back up to look for food. They're amazing birds. We're 1000 miles from land, and these little guys will live out here for most of the year, following the food around in ocean currents. Their flight looks way too energetic, and their wings are sharp and triangular, like a dart, making them inefficient for long travel. To rest, they just settle down on the water and go to sleep. What a miserable roost that must be, I think, looking out at the four-metre seas that have grown overnight. There are whitecaps everywhere in what is looking like an angry and building sea.

# He's growing on me a bit actually. Perhaps slowly like a wart, but I am getting to like the guy

Marty wanders back into the helm. 'The head is ready for business. It was just a broken wire.' Nice one, Marty, I think to myself. He's growing on me a bit actually. Perhaps slowly like a wart, but I am getting to like the guy.

There's a certain tranquillity about *Earthrace* at night: the constant hum of our engines pushing us across the Pacific, the gentle rocking motion as we slide up and over a big following sea, and the sleeping quarters glowing faintly red with a single LED light on. I'm lying in my scratcher nodding off to sleep. 'I had a mate back in New Zealand,' starts Ryan, 'who's able to control his dreams.' It turns out this guy bought a $300 kit which taught him how to 'Lucid Dream', and it included a pair of red flashing glasses he'd wear to bed at night.

I'm pondering the likelihood of this when there's a sudden shift in boat action, as a wave comes in and catches us beam on. *Earthrace* rolls over about 15 degrees then stops suddenly as the port sponson hits the surface. Must be a shift in wind coming I figure, which is weird, because we're right in the middle of the Pacific trade winds. A few seconds later and we're completely airborne, all of us: the boat, Ryan, myself and everything around us . . . and a split second later we crash down in a heap. The bunk above Ryan collapses on top of him and he's clumsily trying to brace himself for the next crash, which we know is only a few seconds away.

I stumble into the helm, hanging onto the rails, as *Earthrace* gets airborne for the second time. Marty is at the helm, intently pushing buttons on the autopilot. I suddenly notice our compass bearing is 110 degrees, or basically east, and we're supposed to be crossing the Pacific in a westerly direction. Marty has an embarrassed look on his face as he glances up, then goes back to the autopilot, hitting the standby button and taking control manually. 'Oh I just pressed the wrong button,' he says sheepishly.

I'd hate to be heading east in this, I think to myself, looking out at the angry seas. These trade winds have been following us since San Diego, and they've gradually built the big four-metre waves we're currently enjoying. But to head back the other way into these waves, as we've just done briefly, would be awkward indeed. It'd be like the Baja bash all over again. Admittedly, at the moment *Earthrace* is low on fuel, plus there is no ballast in the bow, making our short bit of wave hopping even worse.

We're now only about 400 miles from Majuro, a tiny atoll in the middle of the Pacific and the capital of the Marshall Islands, a small group of atolls. I scroll the GPS system over it and scan in. Typical of many atolls, it is basically a rim of land rising just above sea level, with one inlet allowing boats to pass in and out of an enclosed harbour. I'm not sure I'd be buying any real estate there, as global warming and its rising sea levels will probably wipe out many of these low-lying atolls over the next century. Not that I've got two 50 cent pieces to buy any land with right now anyway.

I scurry back down to the sleeping quarters and clamber onto my bunk, thinking about Majuro. People there by our standards are certainly poor, with unemployment running at 80 per cent, and the government employing nearly all the working population. Majuro does boast among the clearest water anywhere in the world, and the diving and fishing here are unbelievable. A pity we won't be experiencing any of it. It's just a four-hour stop for refuelling and maintenance and we'll be off.

It's late the following night before we approach Majuro. '*Earthrace, Earthrace*, we can see you,' a gravelly voice comes in over Channel 16 on the

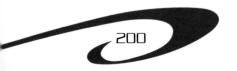

VHF. We're just coming up to the lagoon entrance and are surprised to hear anyone out here. Lagoon sounds picturesque, but in fact the entrance is a cauldron of white water and froth, with 25-knot trade winds sending waves crashing into the tiny atoll. We had just lined up on the channel lights, but this guy is apparently here to guide us through, so we do an abrupt U-turn, back into the four-metre waves to wait for him.

It's an unpleasant halt to things, sitting in these gnarly waves, knowing a lagoon waits just a few hundred metres away. Finally, our friend arrives bouncing up and down in a little boat, weaving his way past us. As we proceed in, he ignores the channel, instead heading straight towards the rocks. 'Captain, are we not going in through the channel?' I enquire. It turns out he has a better channel, but according to my charts it's a rock-infested reef he's guiding us towards. It takes much convincing on his part to coax me into following. At the last minute he does an abrupt turn to port and we

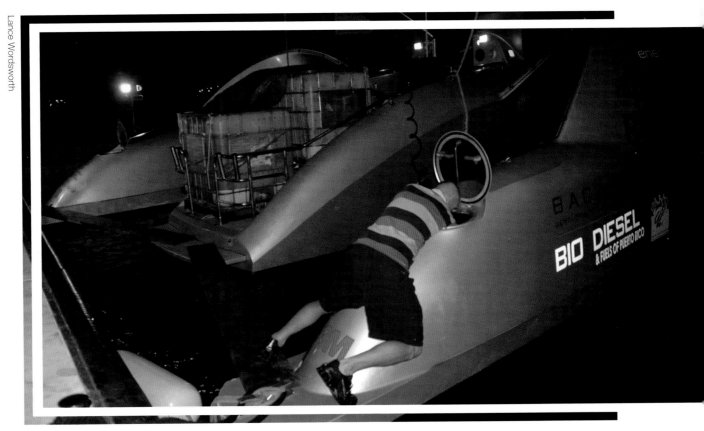

Me bleeding the hydraulics in Majuro (Marshall Islands).

clear around a coral headland that feels perilously close, given the waves still crashing around us.

On *Earthrace*, we feel much safer a thousand miles at sea. These encounters with reefs, atolls and islands always make for a nerve-wracking time, and especially in conditions such as this, where something like a brief loss of power would see us smashed onto corals in a matter of seconds.

An hour later and we're safely docked, locked in among a group of fishing boats, on the island's only floating pontoon. 'So that's what 3000 gallons of biodiesel looks like,' says Scott, peering inside the 20-foot shipping container that was sent from Imperium Renewables. I glance in to see an enormous 1.5-metre-deep plastic bladder almost filling the entire container. Lucky it didn't burst or we'd be in trouble — 10 grand worth of fuel down the drain. The white bladder looks swollen and fat, ready to be disgorged into *Earthrace*.

'You sure it will all fit in dat boat?' asks one of the locals, looking dubiously at *Earthrace*. In many respects this boat is like a floating fuel tank. It almost doubles its weight when going from empty to full, and it drops around 45 centimetres into the water in the process. It is what gives this boat its amazing range. But, looking at it, you do wonder how the fuel all squeezes in there.

# Into pirate waters

Four metre waves are waiting for us as we head out of the lagoon from Majuro. Initially we meet them head on, but as we skirt the island, they gradually swing to a nice following sea as we turn towards Koror. 'Oh stink one,' says Ryan, slamming down the lid of our Qosmio laptop, 'this Skymate system is still stuffed.' He wanders back down into the sleeping quarters and collapses in a heap on his scratcher, with one arm hanging carelessly down onto the floor.

Skymate is a cool system that allows us to send small emails through a satellite system; however, since leaving the US it's been rather ordinary. In fact since Hawaii, some six days ago, we haven't sent or received anything at all. To make matters worse, the system teases us. It says things like 'The system is running' when in fact the only thing really running is a clock. And it shows the odd satellite talking with our system, but never for long enough to get any emails beamed into cyberspace.

I grab the sat phone and have a quick chat to Allison about it, still in Majuro waiting on her flight to Koror. 'I talked to Skymate,' she says, 'and they thought it'd come back online once you pass 175 degrees east.' I look down at our GPS, and disappointingly see we passed that longitude days ago. Stink one alright. My daily blog might be forced into a weekly affair.

I hang up, and the smell of butter, eggs and onion is wafting around the helm. 'Are you sure you don't want some?' Marty asks, as he cracks another egg open and slings it into the skillet. I'd foolishly pigged out on cereal and toast earlier, and have no room left.

'Nah mate, she's right.' Although it's already stinking hot, so I'm not really sure about a hot breakfast anyway.

I glance back at the temperature gauge hanging on the bulkhead. It's already 35°C and it's not even nine in the morning. As we've come south it's been gradually getting hotter. Yesterday afternoon it was up to 41°C, which is not far off our record of 44. Not that we really want to go breaking that record. One reason it gets so hot in here is there is no air conditioner, and with waves like we're currently getting, the front hatch has to be closed. So the result is a hot, sweaty, humid sauna. Or you can go outside and get wet from the waves crashing over us, which at times is the only way to keep cool.

'Beep ba da beep. Beep ba da beep.' Now that's a strange noise I haven't heard before, and I'm trying to figure out what bit of electronics is making it. All quiet now. Was it the GPS? The engine controls? They all stare at me blankly. A lone albatross comes swooping down by us. Amazing birds, just travelling the oceans and covering thousands of miles. The bird follows us for a good half hour, effortlessly gliding above us, and every now and then swooping down to sea level for a closer look at things. Albatross numbers have been drastically depleted in recent years, mainly due to being caught in fishing long-lines.

'Beep ba da beep. Beep ba da beep.' There's that noise again, an odd sound. I glance at the VHF radio and its screen is showing 'Excessive — voltage'. What the . . . ?

I switch the engine controls over to monitor voltage. Both are showing around 14 volts, which is about right for a 12-volt system charging. But something doesn't look right. There is a variation in voltage that doesn't look normal: 13.8, 14.1, 14.3, 13.6, 14.1. Then suddenly it jumps to 15.2 volts. Something is definitely wrong.

*Earthrace* has an alternator on both engines, each putting out about 14 volts when charging. 'The voltage regulator on one of them must be stuffed,' says Marty, looking concerned.

'Let's just take the lead off one of them,' I reply, 'and we'll see which of the two units is faulty. Then we'll run just on the other unit until Koror.' Marty disconnects the starboard one and our voltage drops nicely back to 13.8 volts. The trouble now is we've got only half the charging capacity we had before, so all the non-essential electronics get shut down, which also means no cooking.

# It's stinking hot all day, and we all just sweat, albeit some more than others

'Man something in here travels,' says Ryan, wrinkling his nose up as he clambers down into the sleeping quarters. He's got his holey pair of underpants on, and is sporting about four inches of plumber's crack. He's also just been outside for a wash in the salt spray, so he's probably the only one who doesn't smell, although his holey undies have done a few rounds since their last wash. Ryan is right, though. There is a definite blokey smell about *Earthrace* now, and it hasn't smelt this bad since the Pacific crossing last July. It's stinking hot all day, and we all just sweat, albeit some more than others. As a result, our clothes, beds, seats and anything else we care to touch end up covered in sweat and, in the tropical heat, start to pong. To make matters worse, we've turned off all the fans to save power, as we're now running on one alternator.

I wander outside to get some fresh air. The waves are a bit smaller today, maybe only a metre or two in height, but it doesn't stop the tops of a few rollicking over the top of *Earthrace* and drenching me. I wasn't planning on getting wet, but I may as well just soak it up I think, resigned to having a salt shower.

After half an hour I dry off as best I can with my sweat-soaked towel, and climb back through the hatch. The smell of sweating men hits me as I reach the galley. Well, I guess the Customs people in Koror will get a surprise when they board us tomorrow.

I look over at Marty who is staring intently at the engine panel. 'Something's not right Pete,' he says, as he scans the parameters. 'Can you feel that vibration?' I sit there for a few seconds concentrating. It feels like a bad cylinder maybe. Or something caught on the propellers. We ease the engines back and go outside. Both props are clear, but there's a large amount of smoke coming out the starboard engine exhaust.

'It's probably just a bad injector,' says Marty, so we get started on replacing them.

Five hours later and Marty and I are exhausted. The engine bay is well over 45°C, and we're both drenched in sweat, with beads constantly streaming down our face. By now we've changed the full set of six injectors, but the vibration and smoke remain. I signal to Marty to go into the helm for a chat and some water.

# Nothing really prepares you for the breath-taking beauty of these islands of Palau

'What do you reckon?' I say to Marty, pulling a bottle of water from the fridge.

'I reckon it's a bad valve.'

'Yeah. Or maybe a bad cylinder?'

'Look, it could be either. I reckon we should get a new head and piston and ring set ordered for Palau, and we'll just run there on one engine.'


'*Earthrace, Earthrace*, this is Neco Marine, Neco Marine.' I recognise Scott's thick American accent over the VHF the following day. We're still a few miles away from Koror Island, with its hills and rocks just emerging in the distance, lit up by the sun now just peeking over the horizon, and it's been a long slow night, listening to the port engine and praying it holds up to get us safely docked.

Nothing really prepares you for the breathtaking beauty of these islands of Palau. They are among the most visually stunning anywhere on the

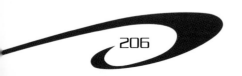

planet, and the slow trip into the harbour at Koror gives us a glimpse of what is the closest to paradise I've ever seen. 'How wicked is this?' says Ryan, looking at a rock precipice above us, with tropical forest hanging out over the edge. Below us the crystal-clear waters reveal an array of corals gradually closing in on us as we enter the channel.

The vice president, the high chief and three senators have all turned up to welcome us in, and they're there waiting on the dock for us as we slide into the inner harbour. There are some brief speeches, followed by a banquet breakfast.

I look around the amazing bar, perched just metres from where we're docked. 'This bar was built for the *Survivor* crew when they were here,' says one of the locals. It seems everyone here has a *Survivor* story, and it certainly made a big financial impact on the place. The TV series had over 350 people living here during filming.

'When do Cummins get here?' I ask Scott, knowing they are a key part in us getting the repairs done.

'Well, Kevin in Charleston has approved the work, but I'm not actually sure when the technician will arrive.' A lengthy discussion ensues about what to do.

'Let's do a compression test,' says Marty enthusiastically. 'At least this would isolate the problem a little.' So Scott wanders off to get one of the old injectors welded into a compression test device.

Sam, who owns an adventure business, invites us over to his bar and yacht club for dinner. We're just enjoying the view, and chatting to some locals, when I notice one of them chewing something. 'What is that?' I ask, pointing at his cheek. His mouth opens in a wide grin, revealing rotten teeth and a dark red liquid.

'Betel nut,' he says proudly, pulling a small packet out of his pocket. They're small green fruit, maybe the size of a walnut. Many of the locals chew these, and it gives you a slight — and legal — high.

He delicately prepares one for me, cutting a half and removing the centre, adding in some lime, and then wrapping it in leaf. 'You put in da corner of ya mouth, and chew slowly.' Which I start doing, but my saliva just goes out of control. They see me swallowing it and laugh. 'No, no, no. You spit.' He leans over the bar edge and spits into the water below. I follow his lead only my hoik is twice as big and twice as red. And for the next 20 minutes, I'm leaning and spitting as the betel nut gradually wears down to a fibrous mass, and my saliva glands get the biggest workout they've ever had. 'And that last piece,' the man says, pointing at my cheek, 'you throw away.'

The following morning we're up bright and early for a bit of adventure. 'Are you sure you want to do this?' It's our dive guide Chad, who we've convinced to take us to a special rock. Ryan and I are standing on a concrete wall built as part of an ammunition store by the Japanese during the Second World War. We're nestled in among lush tropical rainforest, and just over the edge is a 15-metre drop into beautiful blue water. 'If you jump,' Chad continues, 'you cannot tell anyone I brought you here.'

'Yeah, no worries,' we say, trying to figure the best place to jump from, while Lance gets ready to film. Seconds later and I'm plummeting in a mad adrenalin rush, crashing into the water. Ryan follows with a screaming descent, disappearing under water then emerging with a big grin on his

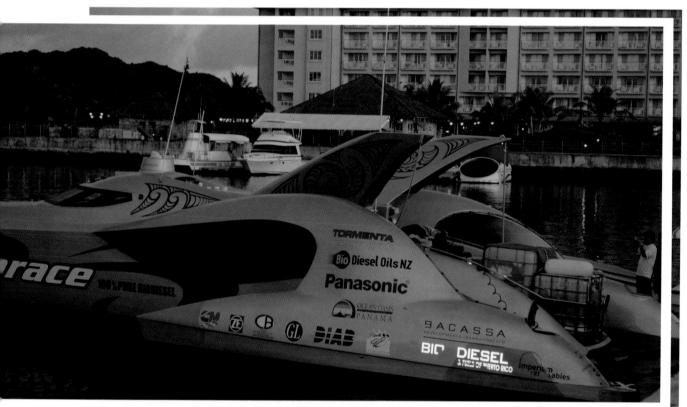

Lance Wordsworth

*Earthrace* docked in Palau.

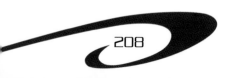

face. We look back up to where we've just leapt from and relish one of the coolest jumps I've ever done. 'Man, it's good to be alive,' says Ryan, still glowing from the experience. This must be the only race in the world where you could take a half day of adventure like this and still have any chance of breaking the record . . . and in fact there's a pang of guilt that we really shouldn't be here. There's nothing I can do on the boat, though, with Marty and Scott sorting what can be done before the spare parts arrive.

A tropical rainstorm thunders down on us as we head over to our next stop, some underwater caves. 'Now, no one has ever free-dived these, but it should be OK,' says Chad, again imploring us to keep it hush-hush. He disappears under water and into a tunnel in the rock face. I give him a minute, take a few big gulps of air and follow. The drop goes down and down, getting darker as you move horizontally under the shelf. I'm starting to wonder if I can find my way back up, and am considering turning around, when I see a small light in the distance from Chad's torch. I follow it along and up, my lungs starting to burn as I surface into an amazing cave.

We tread water and wait for Ryan, who's next. Several minutes pass and no sign of him. I drop down to the first ledge under water to see him swimming frantically towards me, his movements all out of time and rushed. I can hear his throat gulping from lack of oxygen, and I'm thinking he's going to black out, but he comes shooting up to the surface and gulps in a couple of massive breaths of stale cave air. 'That was freaky,' says Ryan, the look of fear in his eyes as he removes his mask. He clambers up onto a rock ledge and sits there shaking. A few seconds later and Allison comes shooting up into the cave.

This is the first of four caverns, all linked by a series of deep underground tunnels. 'There's no way I'm going any further,' says Ryan, clearly shaken by his first descent. So we leave him there in the darkness and continue on through the next three caves, each one getting easier as our lungs get used to the large gulps of air.

Chad shines his torch up to the ceiling of the last cave. It's covered in stalactites. There's a faint hint of fresh air in this last cave, so it must have an exit somewhere. And back out the way we've come, we can just make out a hint of sunlight, winding its way through the tunnel structure. We turn around and head back out, grabbing Ryan on the way.

'You know, this has been one of the coolest days of my life,' says Ryan, as we wash out our dive gear back at Sam's Tours. I look back on what has been an amazing day. We've dived on an old Second World War wreck, jumped off a wicked 15-metre ledge, and free-dived some awesome caves. Not to mention it all happening in the most stunning group of islands I've ever seen. 'Yeah, it's been a wicked day alright.'

We get back to *Earthrace*, where Scott has not had such a wicked day. 'Well,' he says, 'the compression on cylinder one is 1, while all the rest are 24. So cylinder one is definitely stuffed.' We ponder what this all means; that the compression is so low probably suggests a dropped valve or a hole in a piston. Either way, though, it means the head, piston and ring sets Cummins Mercruiser are sending should sort the problem.

'What about the Cummins Mercruiser technician?'

'He should be arriving tomorrow, but when the spare parts will arrive I'm not sure.'

## 'What this means, is we need to drop the sump, remove the piston, remove the cylinder sleeve, and put in a new piston and rings'

Two days later and Joe, our CMD technician, arrives from Guam. Within a couple of hours he has the head removed, and it takes four of us to lever it out of the tight engine bay, over the biodiesel tote and onto the dock. We lie it down like a dead animal. 'Oh, check this out,' says Scott, pointing at one of the valves. A square segment, maybe half a centimetre across, has been blown completely off the valve edge. 'You gotta wonder what caused that?' A few locals wander down to admire our trophy.

We clamber back into the engine bay to check out the piston. Joe and Scott are already in deep discussion. I look down at the piston and shards of metal lie embedded in the top, which isn't so bad. Then to my horror I see the piston is all distorted. A section has actually melted away, exposing the top ring.

'What this means,' explains Joe, 'is we need to drop the sump, remove the piston, remove the cylinder sleeve, and put in a new piston and rings.' Having done this once before on a much smaller engine, I know it'll be a nightmarish job, especially in such a tight engine bay as this. I look over to Scott who's shaking his head in disgust. I'm not even sure we'll be able to drop

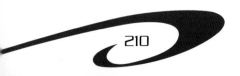

the sump. I look around for someone really small to clamber under and have a look, just as Lance comes wandering back from the dock. 'Lance, you're about to become an engineer. Clamber in under there and see if you can remove the sump.' He looks at me blankly, wondering what exactly this involves. Scott grabs him before he can escape, and seconds later he's disappearing down into the gap between the two engines.

'Well, the good news,' says Scott, 'is all the bits we need are already in the air.' Which is great, but when they'll get here, I have no idea.

Lance starts removing the nuts holding the sump up. 'Hey, what happened with your worms?' I say to him, remembering his drama back in San Diego. Lance stops working and looks up at me with a smile.

'Well, I posted the images on the website, and initially I got a couple of people emailing saying it was a hoax. But then a guy Jefferey from Barbados figured it out. They are the larval form of some kind of fly that lays eggs in meat and cheese. When this is eaten, the eggs will hatch into little larvae that live in your intestines for a while, before coming out your bum and turning into a fly. He reckons I will have picked them up in Korea.'

'And is there a treatment?'

'Nah. They eventually all come out. And in fact it's been almost a week since I last saw one anyway.'

Lance goes back to the sump, reaching in underneath with the ratchet.

I wander back to our hotel Internet room. Allison has a worried look on her face. 'It seems,' she says, 'our parts were not sent after all.' I look down and she's reading screeds of emails from

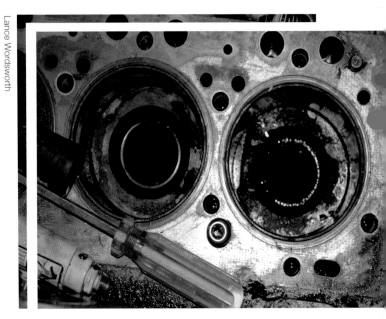

The piston on the left is OK, while the piston on the right has melted.

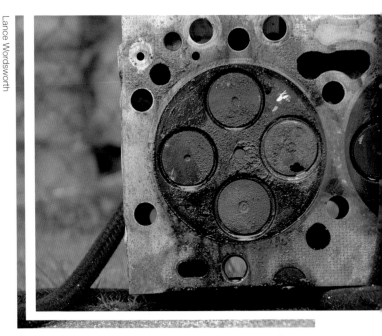

The damaged head, with a hole in one of the valves. The piston started melting, the excess heat of which then caused the damage to the valve.

Cummins Mercruiser, each one unfolding a new segment of the shipment story. By the end of them it appears the head has been sent but not the piston and rings, but she's still not sure.

Ryan wanders in with a big smile, and I give him the news. His smile disappears and he looks out at the harbour just metres from where we're sitting. 'Does this mean we're buggered for the record?' he asks. I do some quick sums in my head. Even if we had a perfect run from here there's no way we'd get the record by Barbados. He sits there shaking his head.

There's also one other thing that's been gnawing at me since last evening. Sharyn had phoned from New Zealand in tears. *Earthrace* has a $70k overdraft with the National Bank, and they're demanding we pay it back now or they'll force us into a mortgagee sale of our house. The trouble is we don't have the money to pay them back yet, and I'm not sure where I can get it from right now. John is working on it, but he's struggling getting

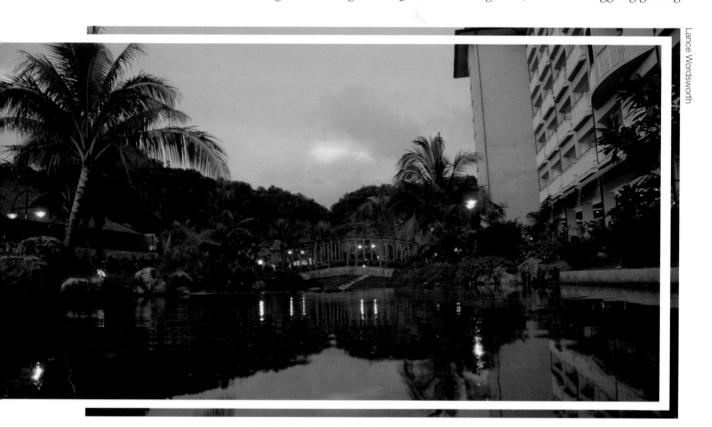

Lance Wordsworth

The flash Palau Royal Resort gave us free accommodation and meals while we were in Koror.

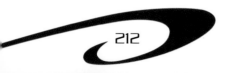

the race money together, let alone another 70 grand. Maybe I should just flag all this and get home where I belong. It's an appealing thought right now.

Scott and Lance also arrive, their faces as long as ours. 'You know guys, it's been a long few days here, how about we go out tonight for a few quiet ones.' The lads all seem keen on this idea. So we start down at the Drop Off bar by *Earthrace* then wander into town. Koror is mostly visited by Asians, and this is evident in their bars, which all seem to sport some form of karaoke. And the people all have their signature song. Some of them are actually quite good. We've stopped at the bar with the most flashing lights at it, and our waitress immediately brings over a bevy of girls to accompany us. 'You buy us lady juice?' they start enquiring. This is a system where you pay a small fortune for drinks that they sip, in exchange for having them sit by you.

The karaoke list is placed in front of us. Some guy is wailing in the back singing an Elvis song and it sounds just appalling. We look through the list and pick song 4888. An hour later and we'd forgotten all about it when the waitress suddenly appears with the microphone. 'You nex, you nex,' she says excitedly. We all look at each other wondering who is going to sing. The tequila by now is starting to kick in so I finally grab the microphone. The music starts and I can hear a few people towards the back of the room singing along already. Some of them here memorise all the songs. I wait a few more seconds, put on my coolest Maori accent, and let rip. 'Wild thing. You make my heart sing eeeeoooow. You make everything groooovy eeeeoooowww.' I don't bother keeping time with the music, and it's more like talking than actually singing, with enough suspect words and made-up lyrics to have the lads shaking their heads. I finish with a flourish. The place is all quiet with a hundred brown faces all looking at us pitifully. 'Ha. How was that?' I say as the waitress takes the microphone from me and scampers off with a scowl on her face. 'Well, I thought it was good.'

The days in Palau gradually tick by. Our replacement head, gaskets, cylinder sleeve and rings arrive, but no piston. We scour the local engineering workshops hoping to find a spare piston but none will fit. Then the guys in Guam locate what they think is the right piston, but when it arrives we find it's for an earlier-model engine and won't work correctly in ours. Finally, after we've been here a week, the correct piston turns up. Within 12 hours it is installed and running and we're back on our way.

'See ya mate,' I say to Lance, giving him a quick *Earthrace* handshake. 'Watch out for those worms.' All the ground crew are there to see us off, no doubt relieved that the repairs are done and we can finally get on our way to Singapore. Things took so long in Koror that it has certainly ruined our chances of getting the record by Barbados. And I'm still in trepidation of what will happen next.

'All clear,' yells Ryan, as the ropes are pulled in and we exit the dock. Half an hour later and we're gradually getting up to speed, the reef, and hopefully Koror, all behind us.

'Hey Pete, check this out.' Hedley, our new engineer, is driving and he's got another unusual vessel for me to look at. I grab the binoculars and look out to starboard, where there's a small trimaran, seemingly drifting aimlessly. It's one of the weirdest-looking boats I've ever seen. A low central hull made of steel, with two outriggers connected by curved beams, and a little wooden cabin perched on top.

# We have the dubious good fortune of passing through the three worst pirate areas in the world

We're just passing the southern tip of the Philippines, and starting to see lots of boats now, as we head towards the Sulu Sea. I look out to port and there's another one of these canoe-like things we'd been picking up on radar overnight. The strange thing is they've actually put some sort of palm tree on one end, which sticks up a couple of metres. I guess it's so you can see the thing above the waves, but what it is I'm not sure. 'It's a tsunami early warning device,' says Hedley authoritatively. 'This sea is littered with them now.'

Up ahead there's a tanker that we're slowly overtaking. I scan the binoculars towards it and notice plumes of water being pumped down both sides of the clean hull. 'What are they up to do ya reckon?'

'Oh that's anti-piracy measures,' says Hedley. 'It makes it harder for small boats to pull alongside and have someone climb up. Speaking of which, what are our plans if pirates attack us?'

It's a good question. We have the dubious good fortune of passing through the three worst pirate areas in the world — the Sulu and South China Sea, which we're entering now, the Straits of Malacca, which we'll go through after Singapore, and the Red Sea, which will be just before the Suez Canal. 'Well, mate,' I start, 'we have no guns. Our best form of defence is to just outrun them.' I go on to explain that there are several sections of the boat that are bulletproof. The spars, which go through the galley, are the strongest section, and would stop everything bar a .50 calibre bullet. So you can hide behind them if you know roughly where the shots are coming from. You can also hide between the two engines, or in the forward section behind the ballast tank.

Hedley seems unconvinced.

'Are you sure you don't have any guns on board?'

'Look. Pirates are after a free and easy lunch. They want fat-cat boats that they can board easily, ruffle the passengers up a bit with no hassles, and wander off with a bit of cash and jewellery. Or take a couple of hostages. Now does this boat look easy to take? It's hard enough boarding it while stationary, let alone at 30 knots. And does this boat look like a free lunch?' Hedley ponders this a few minutes, looking out to the tanker now immediately beside us. 'And who's driving while all this is happening?'

'I'll just put her in autopilot and hide with you.' Hedley smiles, and goes back to looking at the tanker.

The sea is oily flat by now. The smoothest we've seen while on the entire race. I leave Hedley in the helm and head up to the roof. Ryan nods and smiles as I sit down against one of the horns next to him. 'Wicked day, eh,' he says, putting his book down and looking towards a small island we're about to pass. There are small huts along the beach of what looks like a sleepy fishing village. 'Did you know there are over 7000 islands in the Philippines?' he asks, now scanning the shoreline with our binoculars.

We sit silent for a while, just soaking up a gorgeous morning. Then Ryan mentions our situation in the race, which has been nagging us since Koror. 'If we have no chance of getting the record by Barbados, why don't we just quit in Singapore?' Of course, this is one of our options. We could also continue on to Barbados and stop there, finishing the voyage at least.

'There is another possibility,' I reply. 'We could continue on, even as far as San Diego, which would give us a fighting chance of the record. We don't have to just finish in Barbados. We can choose any start or finish point we like, and San Diego would wipe out all that lost time in Panama and Guatemala.'

'That would mean that in Singapore, instead of being half way through the race, we're not even a third through it,' he says dejectedly.

'Yep. But at least it gives us a chance to deliver what we said we would.' He sits there for a few minutes looking back at the island. The trouble with going on to San Diego is we have no logistics or fuel organised, no funding, and a team that is increasingly jaded from the ordeal we're going through.

'Hey Pete, we've got company.' It's Hedley yelling from the helm, and he's picked up a boat on radar zooming directly towards us. I get the binoculars out but cannot see anything, although the radar still puts them four miles away. Nothing to worry about, I assure everyone. But in the back of my mind I'm uneasy.

It seems a strange path for them to take, on a direct collision course with us, and with nothing past us that seems like a natural destination. A few minutes later and the radio squawks: 'Erice, Erice, dis wa-ship, wa-ship.'

'Do you think he was calling us?' I ask the lads, now all peering out to sea.

'There it is,' says Hedley excitedly. Out of the gloom comes a big grey catamaran, not a pretty boat, but certainly a decent little patrol or fishing vessel. I grab the binoculars and check it out. Too flash for a pirate, I think to myself. Must be military, although there are no markings on it.

'Erice, Erice, dis wa-ship, wa-ship.' The radio squawks at me again. I grab the handpiece and reply 'This is *Earthrace*, are you calling us?'

'Yes. Yes. Dis warship.'

There follows a strange conversation where we understand so little of what they're trying to say, other than they are a warship, and they want to talk with us.

'We are going to Kota Kinabalu to clear Customs. If you would like to board us please meet us there,' I reply, not knowing if they understand or not. The boat cuts in behind and follows us at a distance of about 100 metres, a .50 calibre machine gun staring at us menacingly from their bow. Ever since the Colombian navy shot at us last year, I've been very wary of military vessels.

We cut in close to the coastline and a chopper buzzes down beside us, a cameraman hanging precariously out the door. Well, they won't try anything with cameras rolling, I think to myself.

Half an hour later and we're pulling into Sutra Harbour in Kota Kinabalu, the capital of the Malaysian state of Sabah. There on the dock are around a hundred people to greet us, including some warriors, dancers, dignitaries and media.

We scamper ashore, blown away by the reception. The Minister for Tourism and several other government officials come forward with gifts. Ryan is shuffling around with his camera getting footage, while Hedley looks on shaking his head in disbelief.

'How cool is this?' I say to Ryan, as a warrior comes up and offers me a shield and machete.

'Did our navy escort you in OK?' enquires one of the ministers.

All too quickly we're packed up and leaving. What a wonderful introduction to Malaysia I think, as we pull away from the dock. I reckon I'll come back here one day with Sharyn and the girls. Mount Kinabalu disappears behind us as we head back out into the South China Sea.

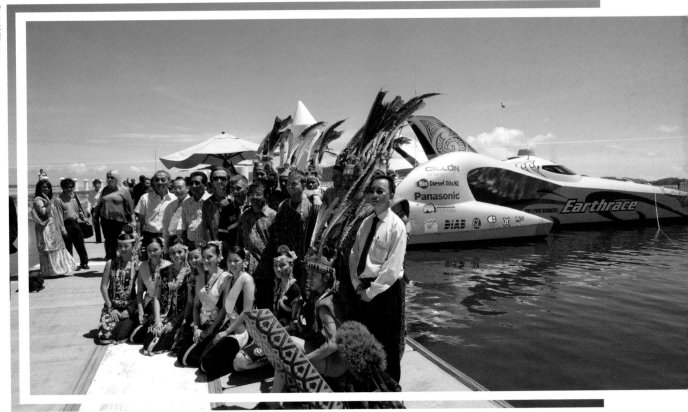

Dale Williams

It was an amazing group of warriors, dancers and government officials who greeted us when we arrived in Kota Kinabalu (Borneo, Malaysia).

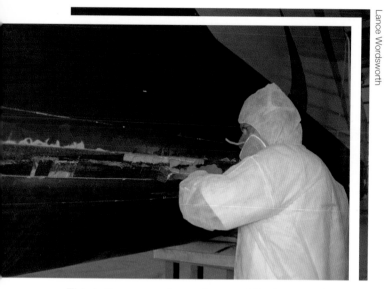

Lance Wordsworth

This is the gouge from when we hit a log near Borneo. Damage went through the Kevlar, carbon and foam, but thankfully did not quite get through the inner skin and fuel tank. We did a quick underwater repair in Singapore using Splashzone, then pulled *Earthrace* from the water after the race to do a full repair.

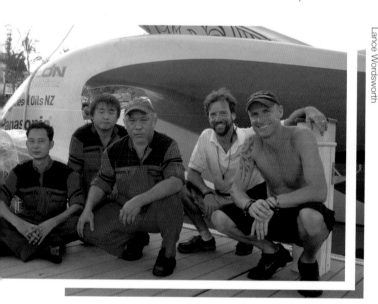

Lance Wordsworth

The Cummins Mercruiser Diesel team in Singapore with Scott and myself.

There's a dull thud as we run something over in the water. Hedley is driving and looks startled. 'What was that?' he asks.

'Well, you're the one driving,' I reply, somewhat disappointed he didn't see the object before we hit it. Half an hour later and there's another dull thud, this one louder and heavier than the last. I scramble up to the navigator's seat for a look. All around us are twigs and branches in the water, most of them relatively small, but the odd one big enough to do some damage.

'Oh, check that out,' says Hedley, pointing in the distance. I grab the binoculars and look at an enormous tree lying with its stump end sticking out of the water. It's at least three metres across, and would easily sink us if we hit it.

One of the locals had warned me about this earlier in the day. Fishermen tow logs out to sea, and they form aggregation devices, attracting fish from all over the place. The trouble is they are a major risk for boats, especially lightweight race boats like *Earthrace*. We spend the next two hours dodging logs and branches, our track resembling more a yacht tacking than a powerboat. As light starts to fade, it seems, thankfully, we're through them.

At 1.30am we're suddenly all woken with the horrendous sound of splintering carbon, followed by some dull thuds. I grab the torch and start looking through the various underfloor sections and through the engine room for leaks. Nothing coming in, but it was a big blow.

'It could have ruptured the fuel tanks,' I say to Hedley, who is sitting there looking petrified. We isolate the main and day tanks, and check the water traps on the Racor systems, which all

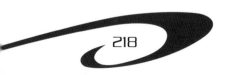

seem fine. 'Let's just run at 10 knots for a while, and keep a close eye on the night vision system.' It's a long slow night and we make painfully slow progress as we head towards Singapore.

By the morning we're back up to speed, and Hedley comes up to me looking serious. 'Actually Pete, I'm going to leave you guys in Singapore.' It comes as a shock. We flew him to Koror at considerable expense, on the understanding he'd be with us for a month, and now he wants to bail out after just one leg.

'What makes you want to do that?' I reply, trying to understand his motives. He was pretty scared, like we all were, after we hit the log last night. But I didn't think it was enough to make him quit.

'The bilge. It's a fire hazard,' he blurts out.

'Well, you're the engineer, mate. Why didn't you fix it in Koror before we left?' I spit back at him, angry that he'd pull such an excuse. He shuffles his feet and looks away.

'There are lots of reasons, really. This just isn't my kind of thing.' I can tell he's made his mind up, so I don't bother trying to convince him otherwise. The last thing I want is people aboard who don't really want to be here.

I beam an email off to the ground crew, requesting they find us another engineer. With a day's notice, though, it'd be a miracle if they manage to find anyone at all. What is it about these engineers? Marty lasted three legs before he quit, and now we've only had Hedley for a single leg. Or maybe I'm the problem. Am I asking too much of these guys?

The following morning we're docked at the prestigious One Degree Fifteen marina in Singapore. I'm not sure if the person who came

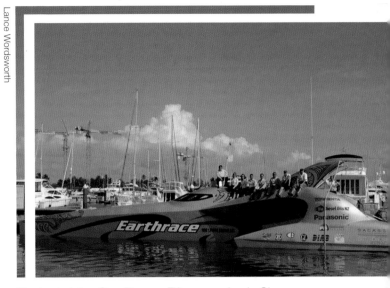

Docked at the One Degree Fifteen marina in Singapore with our sponsors. Note how low *Earthrace* is in the water when fully fuelled.

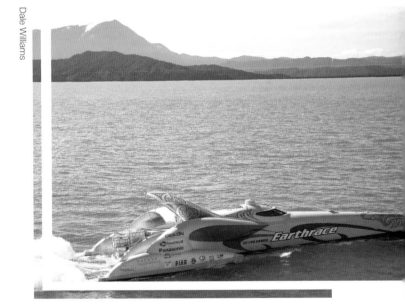

Coming along the north coast of Borneo, with Mount Kinabalu in the background. Fishermen in this area drag logs out to sea to attract fish, but many boats then hit these and get damaged.

up with the name is a marketing genius or a klutz, but it sure is a swanky place. They've generously given us accommodation, docking and press facilities while we're here. It's a member-only compound, and it seems more like a country club than a marina.

Our full team is here, and we gather together for a meeting. 'Right, we need to figure out if we are going to continue with this race, and if so, we need to find a replacement for Hedley.'

'And we need to find some money,' interjects John. 'We have none left.'

Everyone quickly agrees on having our start and finish changed to San Diego, instead of Barbados, which gives us a chance at the record, although with the week we lost in Koror it is still a difficult challenge. The fuel and funding to achieve this, however, is not easily sorted.

'How much money do we have?' I ask John.

'As things stand today,' he says, we have only $1400 left, which will get us to India but no further. There's also this 70 grand to stop your house in New Zealand being sold. I just don't know where we can pull that sort of money at the last minute like this.' We sit there for a few minutes, tossing around ideas.

Ryan sits up and starts talking. 'We just need to have faith. And we need to just keep knocking on doors and asking people to help. We've been in this position many times, and each time it looks like we're buggered, someone always comes in at the last minute to bail us out. Remember before the race we had no money, and we were talking of giving up, and then in those last two weeks we got that big chunk of money from Ciclon in Puerto Rico, and then another 50 grand from Bacassa in Barbados.' He sits there looking around the team, who are all silent.

John gets a smoke out and lights up. The stress of all this seems to affect him more than most, as he's the one charged with raising the funds for us. 'What about a replacement for Hedley?' I enquire.

'There's this young guy Peter from Christchurch in town who's interested,' says Scott, 'and he could leave with you guys tonight.'

'What qualifications does he have?'

'He breathes and he has a pulse.'

We finish the meeting, and get stuck into maintenance and repairs, then load up with fuel.

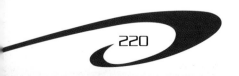

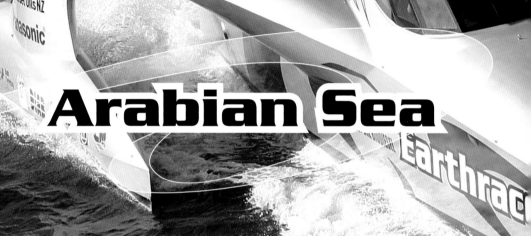

# Arabian Sea

It's late in the evening by the time we leave, now with Peter, our new crew member. To clear Customs in Singapore, you wait on your vessel between two islands and call them on VHF radio. It's after dark before they finally arrive to clear us, and the waterway is getting more and more congested. Finally, our 'zarpe' or clearance document and passports are returned and we're off, but it's into the mother of all traffic jams.

Ahead of us are literally hundreds of boats, in what has recently become the world's busiest port, ahead of Rotterdam. Ryan and Peter are scanning for vessels coming close, while I'm switching between the radar and FLIR infra-red night vision system. The radar especially makes a daunting picture. Each dot, and there are hundreds of them, represents a potential collision, and there are just too many to track them all.

'There's a guy coming up at 10 o'clock,' say Ryan hurriedly. I track him down on the radar, now zoomed right on the boats immediately around us.

'Looks like he'll pass astern,' I respond, although, looking at his path, not by much.

'Ferry coming across our bow soon.' Peter has spotted a small water taxi roaring across our path. We slow to pass behind him. The shipping lane half a mile away beckons on my GPS — a sanctuary of order, relative to the chaos of this traffic jam of random boats. Finally, we make it to the edge of the shipping lane, gingerly picking our time to enter. A big Panamax container ship comes rocking past and we slot in behind her. No one will mess with us here.

# 'Eartrace, Eartrace, dis is Singapore Maritime Pleece, what are your intentions, over?'

Half an hour later, still tucked in nicely behind the Panamax, a spotlight suddenly blinds us. A small boat has been following us from outside the lane for about 10 minutes, slowly edging closer. I grab the VHF to tell them where to go, when suddenly a blue flashing light appears on the vessel. Oops. Let's keep quiet instead.

'Eartrace, Eartrace, dis is Singapore Maritime Pleece,' the radio squawks, 'what are your intentions, over?' The voice has a strong Indian accent, and I'm tempted to say we're off to India where you're from mate, but think better of it. This 'what are your intentions?' we've been asked a lot lately. And I've always wondered exactly what to say. We are going to India? We are on a bearing of 270 degrees, changing to 290 degrees in two miles. We are going to follow this container ship. We're going to blow up a cruise liner. I wonder what'd happen if we said that.

'We are on our way to Cochin in India, and we cleared Singapore Customs and Immigration half an hour ago, sir.'

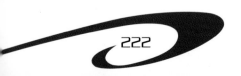

'And what is your boat speed captain?' Now this question is odd. He's been following me for a while now and knows exactly how fast we're going.

'Maybe there's a speed limit in here,' says Peter, 'and he's about to give us a speeding ticket.'

'Um, 17.9 knots, sir,' I reply. There's a pregnant pause on the VHF.

'Vely good, Captain. Have a good voyage.'

We follow the container ship for a couple more hours, then as the traffic lightens up, pull past her and on our way up the straits of Malacca.

We're still some 30 miles south of the city of Banda Aceh on the tip of the Indonesian island of Sumatra, whose waters are the second of three major pirate areas we cross on our voyage. It's 2am, though, and any pirates would be hard pressed to board us in the dark, and especially with the swell now running. Come to think of it, it's odd that we should have this swell rolling down here, as the winds were forecast westerly. Maybe it's the remnants of big waves crossing just above Banda Aceh. That wouldn't bode well for our crossing of the Indian Ocean.

Ryan comes running up into the helm with a startled look on his face. 'Oh, sorry bro. I went to sleep without waking you.' He's been sleepwalking a lot lately, and normally his story is he fell asleep while at the wheel, or went to bed without waking us.

'Nah mate, it's all good. Just go back to bed and I'll wake you in a few hours.' He looks relieved, nods his head and returns to his scratcher. I've had similar dreams and sleepwalking lately as well, although my episodes tend to have us heading for rocks or other boats.

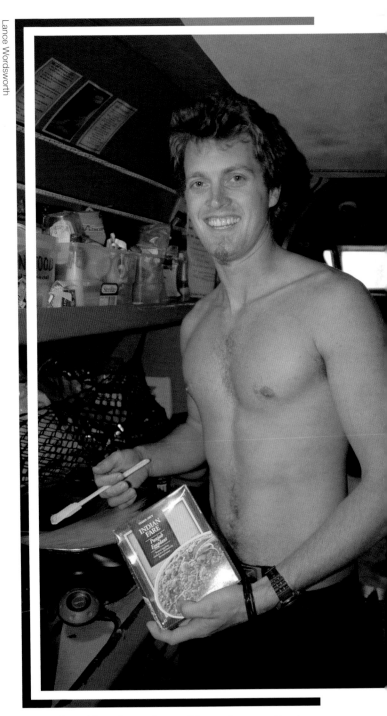

Lance Wordsworth

Ghandi cooking dinner for us. The galley was fine in flat water but got difficult in big seas.

I go down to wake Peter up. He's got a goatee that he's tied up into what looks like a cotton bud of hair, but right now it's got a bend half way down. He's in the starboard pipe cot and lying on his back, which seems to be the only way to get a decent sleep in them. If you lie on your side you get a carbon tube in your knee. Peter doesn't wake up easily. After 30 seconds of shaking him, I resort to the 'torch in your eye' trick. He suddenly blinks awake, and clambers up.

I stay with him for his shift as we pass above Aceh, the troubled province seeking independence from Indonesia. An email came through earlier in the day predicting we would land smack in the middle of the first monsoon of the season, and as we turn west towards India, it greets us. There are 25-knot winds and two- to three-metre waves racing towards us, and it'll be a long battle from here. Our timing to do the record attempt in March and April was largely weather based. It is a short period where the Atlantic and Pacific oceans flatten out, and before the monsoon and hurricane seasons have started. With all the time we've lost along the way, we're now into June, and starting to hit deteriorating weather patterns, which will likely be with us for the rest of the record attempt.

Later that day and the conditions remain crappy. I wander into the helm and scramble into the navigator's seat. These seats are like a sanctuary. They fit snugly around you, bracing you against most impacts, and allow you to rest most of your muscles. 'You know, in conditions like this,' I say to Ryan, who looks up from the book he's trying to read, 'it's just so difficult to do even the most basic thing — like taking a pee.'

'Nah bro, the pissing is easy. It's just getting it on target that's difficult.'

'What about dinner, mate, you cooking?' I ask, hoping he'll whip up something. He's a pretty good cook old Ryan. No meat, of course, with him doing the vegetarian thing, but he's probably made more great meals on board than anyone else.

'Maybe a couple of those ready-made Indian meals. Quite appropriate when we'll be eating there in a day or two,' he says, wandering into the galley and bracing one leg against the starboard spar. He tips the contents of a 'Butter Madras' sachet into a plate, balances it into the microwave, and slams the door shut before it can escape.

A few minutes later he emerges with a steaming plate and hands it over, although there's only about an inch of food left in the bottom. 'Where's the rest of it?' I enquire.

'Oh some went on the door, some went on the bench, a small amount on the floor, and a little was left in your plate if you still want it.' He motions to take the plate back.

'Bugger off mate. I'm not complaining.' A big wave hits us and a glob of boiling hot curry soars off my plate and onto the floor beside me.

'Better eat it quick, Pete,' he says, smiling as he wanders back into the galley to prepare his own.

I look over the bow and a big wave is engulfing us, its breaking top sweeping over the helm in a rush of noise and energy. We drop down the other side with a crash, sending white water out either side, then the next wave starts its relentless drive over us.

'Can you smell something Pete?' says Peter, who's just come back from checking the engine bay.

# There's about a foot of diesel in the forward compartment. It's all through the sea anchor, the drogue, our dive gear

'Nothing but your smelly body,' I reply, but then I have a sniff, and I can smell something. Diesel . . . and yet we're currently running on biodiesel from Malaysia. The only diesel we have is a couple of five-gallon containers in the engine room, and a single 30-gallon container in the bow.

'Check the bow mate. It could be coming from there.' Peter scurries to the front and returns with bad news.

'There's about a foot of diesel in the forward compartment. It's all through the sea anchor, the drogue, our dive gear, power cords, all sorts of stuff.' My heart sinks at the nightmare job this'll become.

We turn *Earthrace* around to go with the waves, and I clamber inside for a look. The single drum of diesel has burst, while the four biodiesel containers remain intact. I decide to clear the biodiesel first, so Peter passes in the 12-volt DC pump and we start transferring from the drums into our main tank. Thinking about it I should have done this on the first day, but I'd sloppily put it off.

By now I'm covered in diesel, and I can feel it eating at the various cuts and sores. My head starts spinning from the fumes, which are almost

overpowering. This I know is real crap diesel, no doubt wreaking havoc among the few brain cells I have left. Peter keeps talking to me ensuring I don't blank out. Half an hour later and I clamber out, desperate for clean air.

We finally transfer the diesel, now just swilling around the bottom of the compartment, into a spare drum next to the anchor, and put a second strap on it just to make sure. The hatch is then closed, sealing in all those evil fumes until we get to India. By now the whole boat reeks of diesel. It's on our skin, in our clothes and through our hair.

'Fancy a swim guys?' I say, wandering out the back with a bottle of soap. The sea actually doesn't look that inviting, though. The waves are big and gnarly, but I'm covered in diesel and keen to be rid of it. I grab a rope on the transom and drop in for a quick rinse. There's a sudden burst of colour all around me from the oily diesel, then it's gone as the next wave rolls on through. I cling to the rope until it's past us then clamber back onto

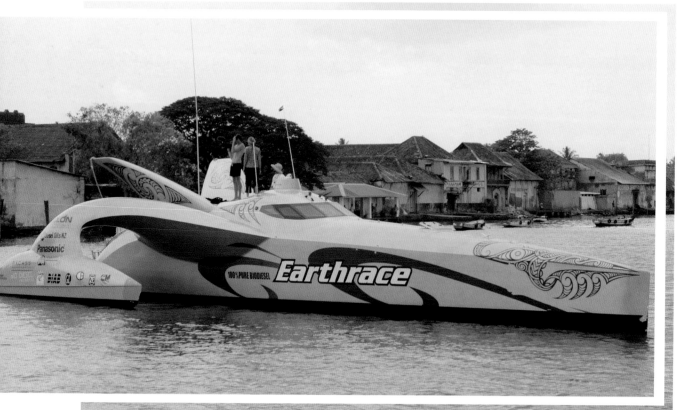

Lance Wordsworth

Cochin, India. This is the filthiest waterway I've ever seen.

the transom. 'Man, this water is nice,' says Peter, just emerging from his first dunking. Dangerous as well. Peter struggles against a series of waves before finally clambering aboard.

Suddenly my body feels awfully tired, but the sleeping quarters are totally diesel ridden. So I drag a mattress up onto the galley floor and lie down. My head spins again, and my stomach starts to send those first little signs that a chunder might be on its way. It would be my first on *Earthrace*. Not for the first time, I wonder if this is really all worth it. But then I've only got myself to blame for this cock-up.

The following day and we're a tired and dejected crew. 'I never slept a wink last night,' says Ryan, climbing gingerly from his makeshift mattress in the galley. The fumes in our sleeping quarters were so bad we ended up in the galley and helm, and it seems we're all nursing hangover-like headaches. Ryan's hair is in all directions, his eyes bloodshot, and he's pale and sickly. It'd be fair to say he's never been a morning person, but today he looks dreadful.

'Did you feel that big wave last night?' asks Peter, suddenly happy to have someone to talk to. Statistically, one wave in every 300,000 is four times the height of the average wave around it. Well, we must've hit one of those last night. After going over and through the wave, we were airborne for what seemed like an eternity, before crashing into an enormous hole. It rattled every screw and bit of composite on *Earthrace*. I don't know how big it was, except that it had to be enormous. At the time the rest of the sea was around three metres, which was uncomfortable, but manageable.

'Yeah I was airborne for ages then came crashing down on the spar,' I reply, 'and I've got a big bruise on my back as a souvenir.' I rub my hand over the tender area. We're all sporting bruises of various sizes right now, mostly resulting from the last three days of monsoon.

Peter disappears into the engine bay, while I grab a torch and start looking over the composite structures for any cracks or delamination. Only a minute later and Peter returns with a worried look on his face. 'Pete. You'd better come see this.' We climb down by the starboard engine and he shines his torch on one of the forward engine mounts. To my horror, one of the bolts that fix the engine to the mount has sheared right off. 'That's not all,' says Peter, 'this one here's gone as well,' pointing his torch at one of the rear mounts. 'And the other one back there is bent in an "S" curve.' We methodically work around the mounts . . . and even the bent one ended up shearing. To my amazement, our starboard engine is currently fixed to the engine bed via a single three-quarter inch bolt.

We drop the load back to just 20 per cent on our starboard engine. I don't want it turned right off, otherwise we'll drag the prop and potentially pull the engine from its current precarious position. I just want a small amount of load to keep things about where they are now.

'Hey Ryan. How far till Cochin?' Ryan looks down at the GPS and makes a few quick calculations.

'We should be there about 2am at this speed,' he comes back, 'although there's an email from the ground crew saying we cannot enter the port till 6.30am anyway. Maybe we should just ease off a little more and time it to get there when they want us.'

'Yeah, let's do it. No point hurrying now.'

We're lucky it happened just before Cochin and not on the day we left Singapore. And thank goodness one bolt held!

The following morning we idle into the harbour at Cochin, picking up our pilot on the way in. 'Just dock over there,' he says, pointing to a spot between two big local boats. It's not ideal but it will do till we get Customs sorted. We tie off and I emerge onto the roof of *Earthrace* for my first look (and smell) of India. There are 50 or so workers on the dock pointing at us and talking among themselves. They're dressed in a variety of outfits: some colourful, some drab and some looking rather eccentric.

'Are any of you guys our agent, or from Customs?' I enquire. Blank faces stare back at me.

A sailing yacht called *Rosa* drifts by, with the whole *Earthrace* team aboard, and three officials with paperwork. I start signing all the forms. And they just keep coming and coming: seven copies of this, five of that, eight of these. It goes on and on.

'What about our shore passes?' I ask the immigration guy who's second in line with his forms.

'Not possible,' comes his terse reply.

'What do you mean not possible? We just want three shore passes so we can go ashore to get spares and start on repairs.'

'I can only issue you a shore pass if you have a seaman's licence. Do you have one of these?' he questions me like he knows the answer.

'Oh yes. I have a yacht master's.' But he shakes his head.

'Captain. Your vessel has come in as a ship not a yacht. For me to issue you with shore passes you must have a seaman's licence. Otherwise you must remain here.'

'What about if I pay you some money?' Maybe he just wants a backhander. He shakes his head again, raises his hand as though the discussion is finished, and disappears through the galley of *Earthrace*.

'Then we will come in as a yacht and not a ship!' I yell at him. He turns and smiles, like he knows he's got me.

'All yachts must moor for 48 hours before entering port. If you would like to come in as a yacht you are more than welcome.'

Our agent comes over and gives me a 'settle down' look. He worked hard to get us in so quickly and he's worried I'll jeopardise things. We finally complete all the procedures, albeit with no shore passes, but with strict instructions that our vessel may not move from here.

# The water even looks dead. An ugly brown with on oil slick on top. Welcome to India

Well, if I'm going to be stuck here I may as well enjoy it. Outside it is warming up already. I wander out into the cockpit and look down at the river. What is that, I wonder, at a big yellow tube-like thing drifting by? It looks like an eel. I poke it with the boathook, and sure enough a big dead eel head emerges, its eyes having been plucked out by seagulls already. Next come a couple of chook wings, followed by a dead seagull, a chook's head, a plastic bag, PET bottles. It's a depressing procession of dead things and litter. The water even looks dead. An ugly brown with an oil slick on top. Welcome to India.

Scott meanwhile is busy sorting the engine mounts. 'We need four bolts about this size. Do you know where I can get these?' He is clear in his questions to the locals, but so far no one has come up with anything remotely looking like new engine mount bolts.

'What about trying the engineers on there?' I suggest, pointing to the big boat docked behind us for a refit. Scott looks at the boat.

'Yeeah,' he says slowly, 'worth a try.' He disappears with one of our broken bolts to see what they have.

As he wanders back along the dock we can see a small crowd of people gathered behind us and pointing in the water. As I look back I can see a bird in the water. It is like a baby vulture, with no feathers around its neck, and it is trying to swim under the dock. It's making breaststroke-like motions with its wings, its head disappearing under water for a few seconds as it does so. It then stops, seemingly exhausted, waits a while, and then starts the action again. 'You know, it's the first live thing I've seen in this river and it's nearly dead,' I comment, as more locals wander over to enjoy the spectacle.

Lance grabs John and the dinghy, and a short while later pulls the little guy from the water. He's got amazingly long talons and a big, raptor-like beak. One of the locals comes over. 'It's an eagle. It catches fish in da water, and sometimes day get wery waterlogged and cannot fly.' We take the bird inside *Earthrace* and put him in one of our large plastic containers. 'Our new pet,' says Ryan. 'I think I'll call him Falcor.'

We're just trying to figure out where to get some fish for him to eat, when Scott returns with a triumphant look on his face. 'Hey check these out,' he says, proffering four bolts that are almost exactly what we're looking for. 'All we need to do is extend this thread a bit with a lathe and we're back in business. They're probably not the right metal, but they'll get you to Egypt where we'll have a new set of mounts waiting.' He's a talented guy old Scott. He heads off to find a lathe.

Meanwhile I go off to sort some shore power. I've just got it going when the local dockmaster comes over. 'You cannot get power from dere,' he says, pointing at my connection into their dodgy-looking electrical box. 'First you must make a request.' He's got that officious look about him that comes from wearing a white coat and a badge. He's short and skinny, with wisps of beard all over his face, and I muse he was probably beaten up at school by other kids.

'Well then, sir, I request that you let us take shore power please.'

'No, no,' he replies, 'You must first write a letter making the request.'

'And who do I write this to?' I enquire.

He puffs his chest out, savouring his moment, 'Why, to me of course.'

'And if I write this letter, sir, will you let me take shore power?'

'Well, that depends on your letter.' He smiles at me, like he's won, and wanders off to see what other evils are happening on his dock. We decide instead to take power from the boat in front of us, hopefully bypassing the dockmaster.

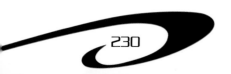

Allison has been watching and shaking her head at the amusing conversation. 'Bad news on the fuel Pete. It's stuck in Customs and won't be here until tomorrow.' Considering the fuel was purchased in Hyderabad, just eight hours' drive away, and not overseas, I'm surprised it has to clear Customs at all . . . and it was supposed to be on dock for us two weeks ago, not arriving the day after we get here. 'We won't be finished the engine repairs until late tonight anyway, so if we get the fuel early tomorrow we'll settle for that.' Allison wanders off, clearly getting frustrated with all the red tape that is an entrenched part of the system here.

With no shore passes, we're faced with another cosy night aboard *Earthrace*. When we arrived in India, we were on target to get the record, despite all the time lost in Palau. A long delay here, however, will hurt us badly. The engine mounts are all sorted with the local Cummins Mercruiser team and Scott having worked all day; now we just need fuel. We head off to our scratchers, hoping for good news on the fuel in the morning.

## My head, neck and back are a mess of itching bites from the onslaught of the last three hours

Zzzzzsssssssssppppppppp. That unmistakeable sound of a mosquito landing on you is universal. And no matter where you are in the world, it plays on your mind. I think it's on my face somewhere . . . or maybe my neck. I yank the sheet up and over, pressing it against my cheeks and chin, hopefully squishing the little bugger. My head, neck and back are a mess of itching bites from the onslaught of the last three hours, the relentless buzzing of mosquitoes making sleep all but impossible.

Thirty seconds later and another mosquito homes in on my heat signature. I scramble up, having had enough, deciding to try to find the insect repellent, which I know is hidden among the first-aid stuff somewhere. My body feels surprisingly drained of energy, and my muscles all ache like I've been drugged — or run over by a bus. It's all I can do to get the three packs of first aid down onto my scratcher before I collapse in a heap, exhausted. Five minutes later and more dive-bombing mosquitoes have me rummaging through the first pack, but I just cannot concentrate. Again I collapse, totally lacking in energy.

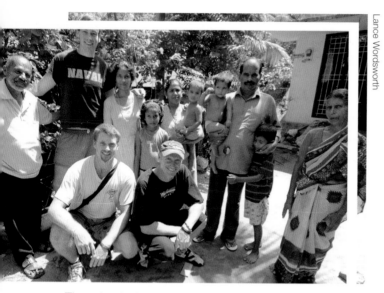

Lance Wordsworth

The tuk tuk driver graciously took Ghandi, Ryan and myself to meet his family. Wonderfully nice and generous people. They had three families all squished into a tiny two-bedroom house. I'm not quite sure where they all slept but it sure would be cosy.

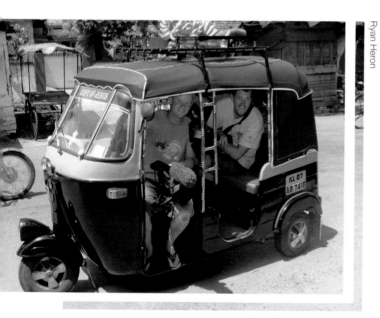

Ryan Heron

Lance and Ghandi in the tuk tuk, on the day we finally left India.

I suddenly have the urge to go to the toilet as my stomach rumbles suspiciously. I drag myself back there, collapsing on the seat with my head on my knees. All hell breaks loose. It feels kind of good, as if I'm getting something evil out of me. But I'm so drained I can hardly muster the energy to move. I sit there resting among the foul stench for a while longer, before finally deciding bed is a better option right now.

The 10-metre walk back to my scratcher takes about five minutes, as I stop half way for a rest, in a heap on the floor. Ryan comes down from the roof, mosquitoes having finally driven him in search of the elusive insect repellent as well. I wonder if he'd heard my effort in the loo a few minutes earlier. 'Any idea which bag the repellent is in?' he enquires. I shake my head and collapse in a heap on my bed, first-aid stuff all around me.

*Earthrace* has an amazing array of drugs and first-aid equipment: a defibrillator, oxygen, saline solution and an enviable hoard of restricted products such as morphine and Valium. Saline saved the life of Gonzales after our collision off the Guatemalan coast. If there's one addition to weight on *Earthrace* I don't mind, it's our first-aid kits. Only now, the entire packs are being emptied around me, as Ryan fossicks among them. Finally, there's a triumphant 'Got ya' as Ryan finds the repellent.

Energy briefly returns as I grab the bottle, spreading it liberally over exposed bits of skin, easily identified from the itchy bites all over them. I fall back against my pillow, unable to sleep, and unable to do anything other than lie there and feel sorry for myself.

'Pete. There's a problem with the fuel,' says Allison, disappointment etched on her face. 'It never made it through Customs last night, but should be here tomorrow.' I look up from bed, having hardly moved in the last six hours, aside from two more runs to the toilet. I couldn't care less about fuel right now, thinking more about my aching body and dodgy stomach.

'Can they guarantee it will be here?' Allison shrugs her shoulders, and heads back out to the galley.

Allison ushers in a half dozen local kids from the Malabar Yacht Club to start cleaning the forward compartments, sleeping quarters and helm, hopefully ridding them of the rancid diesel smell that's permeated *Earthrace*. 'And here's the captain,' she says to them, no doubt pointing at my pitiful body curled up protectively in a ball. They must think I'm lazy, still sleeping at mid morning. But if anything my body feels even worse than during the night. I lie there, eyes closed, while they get to work around me.

A while later and Ryan comes swinging down into the sleeping quarters. 'The fuel is here,' he says, with obvious enthusiasm in his voice. I look out the helm window at the fuel truck, but it slowly edges past us, obviously intended for another vessel. This is like Groundhog Day.

It's midday before Allison returns. 'Bad news. The fuel is still stuck on the border four hours away, apparently with a problem in the paperwork.' There's an element of Chinese whispers going on here. We're just too far out of the loop to know exactly what the status is, and it's costing us dearly in time. Already it is tight for us to get the record, and we're now losing days for no other reason than paperwork and fuel.

'Can we get someone to the border and onto that truck?' I suggest. 'Maybe take Lance and film it, and hopefully they'll be a little more flexible . . . and if we need to pay some money to just make it happen, let's do it.' I think about going myself, but have no shore pass, unlike our ground crew, although I'd be stopping every hour to empty my bowels anyway.

The agent finally agrees to go, but he's unwilling to take anyone with him. It seems they're deliberately keeping us out of the loop. We've reached stalemate with the fuel problem when one of the Cummins Mercruiser guys arrives. These lads would be the hardest-working group of technicians I've ever come across. They just got stuck in and sorted out what was a really difficult challenge, in unbearable heat and humidity. And to top it off, their boss has bribed the right people here to finally get us shore passes. The technician is beaming, holding three precious papers in his hand.

I start thanking him and I notice he's got the most accentuated head wobble I've ever come across. It's not the normal side-to-side Indian motion, but rather a figure of eight. 'Indians often start wobbling when you're talking and they're listening,' Allison had told us the previous day, 'and Cochin is the head wobble capital of India, and hence the world.' It's an endearing habit, one I kind of like.

There's an unusual mix of good and bad here. There are wonderfully friendly and generous people, contrasting with the picky little bureaucrats who do their best to make people's lives miserable, while extracting their own little backhander along the way. Tonight we'll hopefully see more of the former. I clutch the precious shore passes.

The fuel is finally delivered around midnight. However, on testing it, it's found to be dodgy. 'What do you reckon it is?' says Ryan, as I'm holding the little test bottle up to the light.

'Hydroscopic. This fuel is full of water,' I say in disgust.

'Well, can we still use it?'

# We've lost four days waiting here for the fuel to arrive, and when it does, we can't use it

I think about this. The potential of stuffing your engines and being stuck in the middle of the ocean is just too high with bad fuel like this. We'd be doing biodiesel a big disservice, rather than promoting it the way we should be. It's a real shame. We've lost four days waiting here for the fuel to arrive, and when it does, we can't use it. I look back at Ryan and sigh. 'Nah, we can't use this. We have two options. We either call the race off now, or we refuel with normal diesel and continue.'

*Earthrace* has run diesel several times in the past. During initial sea trials around New Zealand we ran diesel to give us benchmark data for comparisons with biodiesel. Also while down south in New Zealand, and up around New York, we ran a blend because of the cooler temperatures. At the moment we have a couple of thousand litres of biodiesel in the tanks, which will give us effectively a B20 blend on leaving here if we add diesel on top. By now the team has gathered around, and we discuss the options. No one is happy about our situation, but in the end we agree to continue.

It's another day before we finally secure the diesel and leave Cochin. We let ourselves down badly here. We should have had someone there much earlier to ensure the biodiesel was delivered on time and that it met specification. Not that we had the funds or resources to do this easily, but hindsight shows not doing so has cost us dearly. When we arrived in Cochin we were on time to get the record, given our revised start and finish location in San Diego. We're now at least four days behind and running out of time.

The monsoon is ready and waiting for us as we head out, but over the following day it gradually eases back. 'What do you reckon about these?' says Ryan, modelling the latest in man nappies from India. It's a golden brown square of material that blokes in India wear. You fold it around your bum then grab the two lower corners, tucking them up into your waist. I have to admit Ryan's looks OK, as far as man nappies go. 'It's really cool Pete. You should try yours.'

Peter, who we've nicknamed Gandhi, because of his man nappies and wispy beard, and who has been wearing his pair since we left India, assures me they're the coolest clothes he's ever worn, next to wearing nothing at all. I wander down into the sleeping quarters where my man nappies have been sitting.

Mine is a drab piece of white linen with a couple of thin blue lines, not like the cool colours the other guys got. How I ended up with the ugly pair I'm not sure. Is it a pair I wonder? I tie the cloth around me but the corners are in the wrong place. I try again and one corner is right and one wrong. Eventually, I manage to get two corners close to where they're supposed to be, and tuck them up into my waist. I pull my undies off and wander up into the helm.

There's this weird feeling you get when you wear no undies. Actually, I'm not sure if Indians wear undies with these or not, or whether Ryan and Gandhi are wearing them. But having them off sure feels good. It feels like the first time I went skinny dipping, the sudden freedom making you think it's naughty. Ryan and Gandhi both take one look at my pathetic white man nappies and crack up laughing. Doh!

I ignore them and plug in my headphones. For a few days now I've been savouring two amazing albums I found buried deep on Ryan's iPod: the latest from Muse, a UK group, and a Kiwi DJ called Module. Both are brilliant in their own way. The Module album especially has a series of awesome tracks to chill out to on night shifts. Playing now is this track about an American who goes into the desert to find himself, which sounds a bit naff, but the song is outstanding.

My mind wanders back to my two girls, who now have their own iPods. Danni, the eldest, told me the other day she likes the new Shapeshifter song. She's showing real promise that girl. Maybe I could take her to a gig or two when I get home.

The iPod drops out and I readjust the cord into the headset, the sounds cutting in and out and then settling back on again. We've had just Ryan's iPod for some time now, after mine was flogged in Palau. Actually, I was amazed that more stuff didn't get stolen there, considering how many people went on and off *Earthrace* unsupervised. Palau seems like a long time ago now. It still hurts that we spent a total of seven days there waiting on the piston, but in hindsight we've only got ourselves to blame. A couple of pistons were originally to be in the spare parts we picked up in Charleston, but they never arrived, and we never followed them up. If we'd had them aboard as planned we'd be in a much healthier position today. The VHF radio squawks, bringing me back to the Indian Ocean. A distant voice, probably speaking Arabic, I think to myself, but too broken to tell.

The following day we pull into Salalah in Oman, which we hope will be a relatively short stop. The big job we've got here is swapping our existing propellers for a new high-efficiency set from Hytorq. I get my dive gear on and jump in, and have only just removed the first two nuts when our agent comes screaming over in his car and jumps out. 'There has been a complaint about you diving. You cannot dive here without a permit.'

'Well, get us a permit then!' I yell back. 'We need to swap propellers and we can't do this without diving.' He looks at me sullenly then drives off, muttering.

We're docked behind a big old freighter, and one of their crew comes over to talk with us.

'I'm Muktah,' he says, extending a wizened hand that's clearly spent many years at sea. I look at the man, wondering where he fits on the boat. He's got a thick bushy beard typical of many North Africans, and his head is half hidden under a beanie. 'If you need something, you ask me.'

'Can you help with refuelling?' says Ryan. 'Just give us a few workers and we'll tell them what to do.'

Seconds later Muktah starts barking orders in Arabic and a dozen Somalis come running down the gangplank towards us. They all disappear into the container with Ryan and start unloading 44-gallon drums.

Lance comes over and we start filming the operation, with Ryan now prancing around in his man nappies getting the Somalis started. Minutes later and our agent returns, again with a flustered look on his face. 'There has been another complaint. You cannot film anything here because you do not have a permit.' I look at him in amazement. The port knew long ago we would be filming here, so it's a bit late to suddenly request we get a film permit. It also seems strange that someone should be complaining at all.

'Well, who has complained?' I ask him. He looks down and shuffles his feet.

'Um. They have.' He points to a military vessel half a mile up the harbour. I look up at the big grey vessel sitting there ominously.

'And who is that?'

'It's an American warship.'

A frown crosses my face. 'Why the hell did you let them in here?'

Our agent doesn't answer, but stands shaking his head like he's embarrassed. If there is one thing that unites the Arab world, it's their hatred of the Americans, not helped in recent times of course with all the bloodshed in Iraq. It must rankle these people to have a US destroyer docked in their harbour. And now the American crew is running around complaining about permits. 'How to win friends and influence people,' I mutter to myself. They'd be better off sending a couple of officers over for a chat and have us as an ally.

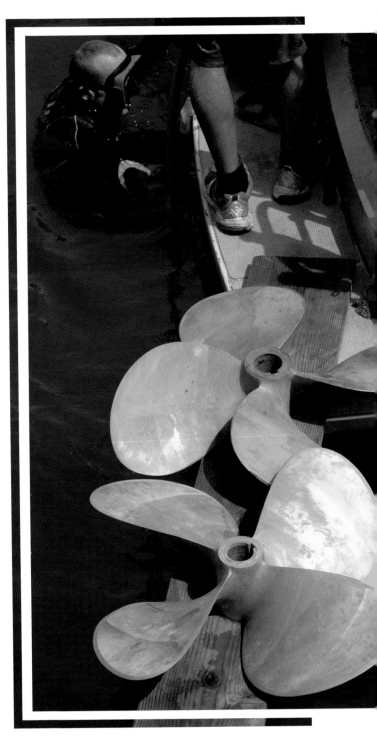

Lance Wordsworth

Me and Ghandi changing the propellers in Oman.

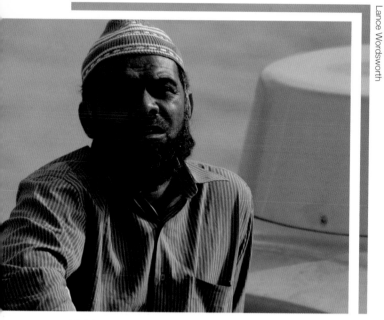

Mukhta helping us with the refuelling in Salalah, Oman.

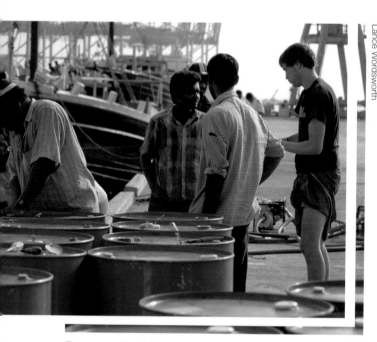

Ryan wearing his man nappies, and getting the Somalis started on refuelling. The fuel pumps are in the background.

I look back at our agent. 'Look. Don't let them win. This is Oman, not USA. You go to the dockmaster and get me a permit to dive and a permit to film and a permit to refuel if we need one of those, and we'll be gone from here in a couple of hours.'

He gives me a weak smile and disappears in his car.

With no diving and no filming, and the refuelling all taken care of, there's not much else to do, so I disappear into the port bathrooms for a shower. It's an open affair with no walls, a row of toilets on one side of the room, and a row of showers opposite. The toilets, though, consist of a small hole in the floor, and a couple of pads for your feet. I remember using these in Libya when I worked there in the oil industry. You squat over them, and it helps if you're a good shot. They also have no toilet paper, instead there's a small water hose with a valve on the end.

I'm busy washing my face when two locals wander in, squatting down on a couple of toilets opposite me. They sit there doing their business, and steal glances over at me every few seconds. How weird is this?

I feel nice and refreshed as I get back to the boat. The permits have arrived, the refuelling is almost completed and Gandhi is busy doing the propellers. John comes running over. 'It's Sharyn for you,' he says, handing me his little Nokia cell phone. 'She's crying.'

'Hello,' I say softly.

'You know how we had to pay that money back to the National Bank or they'd sell our house?' I suddenly have a vision of Sharyn and the girls crying at the house with an auctioneer in front.

'Well, some guy in the States has just transferred back the funds to wipe the debt.' Sharyn is sobbing, amazed I guess that someone could be so generous.

'Who was it?'

'Some guy in Alabama, but he wants to remain anonymous.'

John had apparently sorted this a week earlier. He's grinning from ear to ear as I finish the call.

'Yeah, we've pretty much got the money to finish the race as well,' he says. 'Our website has been going ballistic lately, mostly with traffic to the blogs. Scott put in a plug that we needed funds, and money has poured in ever since, mostly from the US.'

There's an irony in this. We've got the US military half a mile away being a pack of wankers, and yet it is American generosity that is keeping my family and *Earthrace* afloat. I've always believed the US has the worst of many things, and also the best, and this is a good example.

# I've always believed the US has the worst of many things, and also the best

We head back out to sea, our next stop the Suez Canal in Egypt. We have a couple of days of dead flat water, then on the third night, conditions unexpectedly change. 'They just came out of nowhere,' says Ryan, staring intently at the FLIR infra-red night vision screen. It's 4am and all three of us are clinging on in the helm, having been woken by a series of tall breaking waves.

'Ground crew never mentioned any foul weather coming our way,' I reply, still bewildered at how quickly the seas have changed. The clouds part and some moonlight sneaks through, revealing an angry-looking sea. 'Be at least 30 knots I reckon.' There's a loud whoosh as another wave goes seething over us, the FLIR screen going blank for a few seconds as its waterproof lens is smothered in water. We sit there in silence for a while, disappointed at the change in conditions.

Another series of large waves and I'm suddenly aware of a slight vibration. I head down to the engine bay for a look, hoping that I'm just imagining things. To my horror, all four starboard engine mount bolts have sheared off, with the engine now sitting precariously on the mounts, nothing holding it down. These in fact are the same bolts we'd just replaced in Cochin. 'Ryan. Slow her down to five knots and run with the waves mate. Our engine has just become a loose cannon. Peter. Go and grab all the bits of wood and steel you can find.' Peter scurries off to the storage area behind the engine bay and rummages around, while I scrounge up some tools.

The challenge right now is that if we run on only one engine, we will miss our deadline for the canal crossing. But if we run on two, we run a more serious risk of the engine flipping over, or smashing the drive-train to bits. We have to find a way to brace the engine so it can tolerate some moderate loads without moving greatly. Peter by now is back with some wood and steel for bracing.

As the propeller speed increases, so too does the force pushing forward on the engine. With each engine putting out up to 540 horsepower, there is a massive amount of forward pressure. Normally, this force is transferred

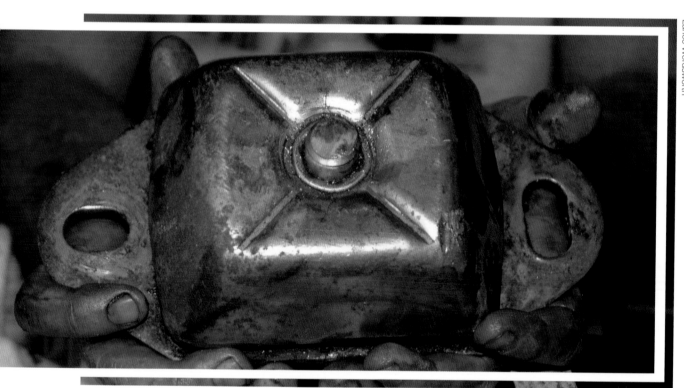

A damaged engine mount. The three-quarter-inch bolt that fixes the engine to the mount has sheared right off. These mounts were just not up to the massive pounding *Earthrace* was subjected to.

through the bolts, into the engine mounts, and from there directly onto the large carbon frame. But right now there is nothing joining the engine to the frame.

There's a large carbon structure right across the engine bay, and only inches in front of the engine sub-frame. 'We'll try to brace the engine frame into this,' I yell at Peter, pointing at the carbon frame. We cut a couple of wedges from the end piece of an old scaffold plank. A two-inch piece of steel box section is braced in front of the port side of the engine sub-frame and then the first wedge is hammered between the two. On the port side we use a large piece of eight-by-two-inch wood and the second wedge.

'Put the port engine in gear, Ryan.' There's a sudden clunk as the engine jolts forward a few millimetres, now pushing against our dodgy-looking framework. Gradually, we load up the engine, and it sits nice and squarely against the frame. We swing *Earthrace* back around into the waves, loading 40 per cent on the starboard engine and 75 per cent on the port. The first few waves come crashing over us, and the engine sits tight.

'Will it last till Suez?' Ryan asks, any thoughts of a nice flat leg with no dramas now shattered.

'Well if it does,' I reply, 'we'll make our canal crossing OK, and if it doesn't, I reckon we're screwed.'

We pull into Egypt with 50-knot winds howling around us and the port and canal closed. Allison has arranged a small dock where we can clear Customs and get the new engine mounts installed. It's after dark by the time we tie up and start work.

'Hey Pete, check that out,' says Allison, pointing at a scuffle between two Egyptians on the dock. There's a small guy in red who's been helping with groceries, and a larger guy who's providing security, although who to exactly I'm not sure.

'What are they fighting over?'

'Apparently it's over the bribe money we're paying, although who's getting what I don't know.'

Baksheesh and bribery are just a normal part of life here. 'If you can look after me, I'll make your boat smaller than it really is,' the measurement guy had said to me half an hour earlier. Fifty bucks later and *Earthrace*, on paper at least, is smaller and lighter than she's ever been, which reduces our canal fees. And we now have his guarantee we'll make a special crossing through the Suez Canal on our own, without the need to go in convoy. This is fantastic, as the convoys are limited to just eight knots. Also the next convoy doesn't leave until 10am the following day, whereas we've just been offered 4am, the time we wanted. There is a catch, of course. Actually, there are two of them at US$60 each, for the two pilots. Cheap at half the price, when I think how precious each hour is to us right now.

'Perhaps to complete this deal,' the measurer had finally said, while looking up at our sat phone, 'you have a spare cell phone I could have.' I explain that our sat phone costs US$6 per minute for calls, and we need it to contact our ground crew. 'Perhaps then,' and he pauses for a few seconds, 'you have some spare electronics.' I explain that we have nothing spare because *Earthrace* is a race boat. He stands silent for a long time, looking around our Spartan helm. I scuttle down into the sleeping quarters and grab him a signed DVD. He looks at it like it's a dead fish, then just as I'm about to throw it back on the bunk he snatches it from me. 'The pilot will be here at four,' he says, smiling suddenly, and shaking my hand.

Sure enough our pilot arrives right on cue. Scott and the three Cummins Mercruiser technicians have just finished replacing the engine mounts. Our food, water and supplies are all loaded, passports stamped and clearance papers issued. A quick clean of the windscreen and we're off, the pilot immediately indicating he'd like 15 knots please. Wahoo: 15 sure beats eight.

The canal is one of the great transport wonders of the world. It saves billions of dollars annually in transport costs, linking Europe with Asia. It has no locks or chambers like the Panama Canal but is rather just a single stretch of water about 200 kilometres long and 150 metres wide.

'We were told this would be in order,' says Ryan, handing the pilot his $60 just before he disembarks at the half way mark. He counts the money and scowls.

'This is not enough,' he demands suddenly, glaring at Ryan. We fossick around and come up with another $10, conscious we still need US$60 for the second pilot. He finally accepts our $10, realising perhaps we have little else to offer. Not before making a request for cigarettes and chocolates, though.

The Chairman of the Canal Authority makes a surprise visit as we offload our first pilot. 'We would like to offer you these gifts,' he says, handing over commemorative coins in delicate cases. We would like to thank you for using our canal, and we wish you safe passage on your voyage. I suddenly feel cheap for not having any gifts available.

'I'm sorry, sir. I have nothing to offer in return, but I guarantee we'll make sure we show the canal in our TV series. He smiles, reminds me there's no filming allowed in the canal, and hurries off.

Just over an hour later, we cruise into Port Said, one of the most famous and historic ports in the world. It's a melting pot of ancient and new buildings, beautiful mosques and water taxis. One of our sponsors has requested we stop in front of their building for photos. Unfortunately, it's also in front of the water taxi and ferry terminals, and there's sudden chaos as we clog up this transport hub while their photographer urges us to stay.

# I look down the dead-end channel, wide enough for us to enter but certainly no way to turn around

A police patrol boat lurches out as I decide to exit, signalling us into a small channel. I look down the dead-end channel, wide enough for us to enter but certainly no way to turn around. To make matters worse there's a 10-knot breeze across the channel, so I might get in, but it'd be a small miracle if I managed to get back out without hitting one of the many little boats tied off in there. I quickly radio our pilot/photographer boat, and they come to our aid, intercepting the police boat. I idle gently past them, the policeman finally signalling us to leave. No doubt for a few bucks from our sponsor.

I gradually inch the throttle forward, and by the time we reach the main shipping channel we're at 20 knots and into the Mediterranean for the first time. 'Can you believe how many people we had to pay off there?' says Ryan earnestly, as he takes over the helm. In total we must have made about a dozen different payments, totalling around five hundred bucks. But we got to enter the canal at the time we wanted, plus we got to exceed their eight-knot speed limit for practically the entire voyage. All up, not a bad deal.

'You know Ryan, I kinda like the system.'

# Last legs

It's a beautiful sea that greets us as we head into the Mediterranean. 'If only it was like this for the whole race,' says Ryan, looking out at the gentle half metre waves rolling in. We're heading almost directly into a gorgeous setting sun.

'Watch for the green flash,' Gandhi reminds us, just as the sun dips below the horizon. None of us sees the flash, but we do witness a stunning sunset. For the last month or so we've been heading west almost continuously, so we've seen many sunsets, but no sunrises — not from the helm at least.

'Hey, does my back have any itchy bites on it?' asks Gandhi, turning around and facing away from us. His back is inflamed with welts and bites. Some of them he's clearly been scratching and a few others I'm sure he'd like to. My back has also been itchy of late. I keep rubbing it against the handle on one of the bulkheads to satisfy the urge. It's a strange satisfying sensation temporarily, but then the bite normally gets worse from the aggravation.

'What do you reckon is causing it?' Gandhi asks, trying to scratch a little spot just out of reach on his back.

'I reckon you've got fleas,' I say jokingly. I then remember the warning about bed bugs. Their eggs are often found in cardboard, and a few weeks ago we had a few cardboard boxes on the floor of *Earthrace*. In fact, some of us ended up sleeping on them through the monsoon in the Indian Ocean when the sleeping quarters were doused in fuel.

'If it is bed bugs, how do we get rid of them?' Gandhi asks, clearly keen to be rid of the pests. We decide to get new sheets and pillowslips at the next port, and to make sure we swap them for clean sets at each port thereafter. 'And we all get to have a nice hot shower?' Gandhi asks. Showers are probably top of the list in terms of luxuries we miss.

I look down at the scabs on my knee. It's been two weeks and they still haven't healed properly. The heat, humidity and lack of showers keep them infected and sore. 'Yeah, mate. I reckon we'll all get showers at the next few ports.' I grab the first-aid kit and start scrounging around for some antiseptic cream to put on my mangy-looking scabs.

'Oh, you look like a leper,' Gandhi says, noticing for the first time how bad my legs have become.

'Oh thanks, bro.'

The following day and conditions gradually deteriorate. Bob McDavitt at MetService in New Zealand has been giving us storm warnings, and we're all nervous at what lies ahead. 'These waves are getting pretty big, bro,' says Ryan. It's not like I need him telling me. I've been bouncing around in my bunk for the last hour and have finally given up trying to sleep. It's mid afternoon and we've just passed Malta in the middle of the Mediterranean. As we've headed out into the current, the seas have gradually built in intensity, now reaching perhaps five metres in height.

'This don't look good,' Scott had responded when we finally reach him from our sat phone. 'There's a great big low, headed right for ya, and you're in for some brutal seas tonight.' This is kind of what I'd expected. I can hear him tapping away on his keyboard as he accesses Bob's various forecasts.

'It seems,' and he pauses, 'you will have a slightly better run if you keep as south as possible against Tunisia and Algeria. The worst of the storm will then pass to the north of you.'

I put the phone down, relaying the storm news to Ryan. 'You know,' he says, 'this is the fourth leg in a row where we've had a storm hit us.' I'd been thinking about this last night. For the last 9000 nautical miles, every wave we've had has been on the nose, not a single following sea since the leg to Koror, which is likely a result of being too late in passing through these waters. We were planning on finishing the race in late April, and by now it's the end of May. Weather is really frustrating; there is nothing you can do about it.

We turn slightly to port, heading straight for Tunisia. There are strong currents against us as we cross the stretch of water, which will make the waves worse for a while, but hopefully they'll abate once we get across.

Brian, who has joined us for this leg, clambers into the helm. It looks like a drunken weave as he struggles with the violent motions. His face is pale and he looks sick. 'You eaten anything yet?' I ask, but he shakes his head. He's now on his third day with us and he's hardly eaten a thing, initially because he was suffering from a stomach bug he picked up in Egypt. He grabs a bottle of water and collapses on his bunk. 'At least you're losing weight,' I suggest. 'Welcome to the *Earthrace* weight-loss programme.' Brian doesn't smile. He just lies there, bouncing up and down as the waves roll on.

The following day and Brian looks even worse and informs us that there was blood in his urine. It probably means his kidneys are bruised, unsurprising really with the punishing waves that have beaten us up for the last couple of days. Brian has fared worse through this storm, as he's spent most of his time in his scratcher, bouncing up and down.

'Maybe we should get you further aft in the boat to reduce the impacts,' I suggest. He lies down in the galley, and I throw him some memory foam and a pillow. The good news is the waves are now abating, and we'll be in Malaga in the morning, where he can get medical attention.

A yellow bulb suddenly lights up on the dash for a few seconds then turns off. I can't make out which bilge pump it is linked to, so I sit there watching, hoping it doesn't come on again. Two minutes later and there it is again, the forward bilge pump is coming on. Alarmed, I grab a torch and run forward, poking my head down into the bilge hatch.

Water is squirting in around the depth transducer, which is mounted into the bottom of the hull. I can see a large carbon plate over it moving up and down as we hit waves, no doubt gradually cleaving open the cracks. I run back to the helm, slow down to 10 knots, and change angle a bit so we're not hitting the waves directly head on.

I sit there pondering the situation. If the plate gives way, we'll suddenly have a gaping wound filling with water, and potentially this would be more than the bilge pump could handle. There are also cracks well forward of the initial area of damage, and if these keep propagating, they'll pass into the fuel tank, which will probably have us dead in the water. I decide to go aft and fill the day tank from our main to ensure we have enough good fuel to at least reach Malaga.

Ryan senses the slowing in speed and wakes up. 'Everything OK bro?' he asks, poking his head around the corner.

'Nah mate. We have a leak.' He clambers up and I explain the damage in the forward section.

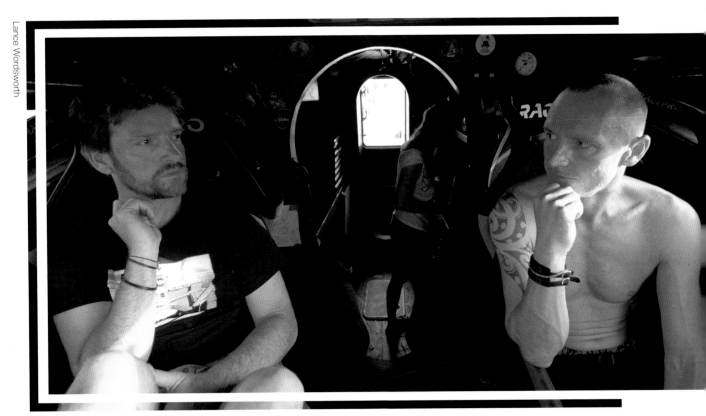

Lance Wordsworth

Scott and I discuss our options to repair the damaged hull.

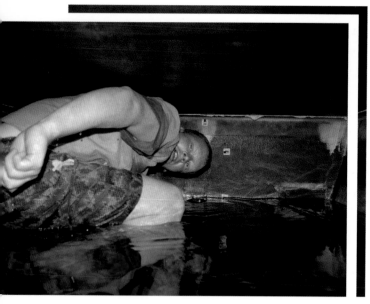

Lance Wordsworth

Adrian Erange, who joined us on the last leg, checking out the leak. It was a scary experience to see water billowing into the hull like this.

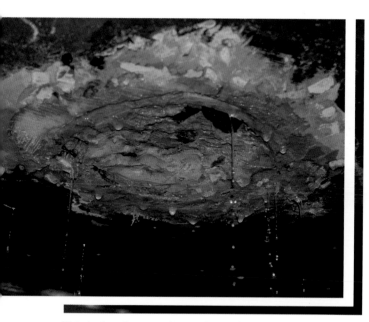

Lance Wordsworth

This is the damaged transducer / hull section after *Earthrace* was pulled from the water. You can see where water is leaking back out from around the transducer.

We sit in silence for a while. 'What about the race?' he finally says.

'Don't know, mate. Depends on how easy it is to repair. But at this stage it sure doesn't look good.' I almost feel sick with despair. It seems every day we have a battle on our hands, and it is slowly grinding us down. But so far we've always dealt with these problems, albeit often losing time. But a boat that leaks is something new for us, and a prospect that fills me with dread.

A wave suddenly crashes into us, and I wince, imagining the plate suddenly giving way. I slow down a further couple of knots. Normally we'd be cracking through these at 20 knots, but here we are at six and I'm worried sick. Just make it to Malaga OK and we'll take it from there.

Early the following morning it's an anxious-looking ground crew that greet us as we clamber ashore. Grabbing the goggles, I swim under for a closer look at the damage. The area around the transducer is fine, but the transducer itself is now recessed higher into the hull than normal, maybe by as much as 10 millimetres. The small crack around it is allowing water to seep in. I give the transducer a push and it lifts up, maybe another five millimetres, as the carbon plate inside flexes. This sure doesn't look good.

Back on the dock, we get the team started on one last-ditch repair effort. Gandhi grinds the area around the transducer away to reveal fresh carbon, while Scott mixes up Splashzone. This ugly brown goo is handed down to Gandhi, still in the water, and he forces the filler liberally into the cavity surrounding the transducer. We apply a similar amount on the inside of the transducer, which by now is sealed.

'What worries me,' Scott says, 'are those,' and he points at the cracks that have propagated a metre forward of the initial damage. 'All that area is now weakened, and will be flexing with every wave you guys hit from now on.' I start poking and prodding along the cracks. In several places the carbon flexes down, the foam underneath having collapsed. In one area the foam has gone completely, and I can see the carbon of the outer skin.

I wander outside to be alone for a few minutes, thinking about our situation. Amazingly, if we continue from here with the speeds we've averaged on the last two legs, we'd actually get the record by about a day. To repair the damage properly, though, we need the boat pulled from the water, and we'd lose at least three or four days, eliminating any chance of the record.

'Let's do this,' I'd said to a weary-looking team. 'We brace the zone as best we can, and we head to the Canary Islands. If the repair holds to there, we'll then look at the forecast for the next leg and make a decision as to whether we continue or not. And if a tropical cyclone or storm looks at all likely at any time from here, we abandon the attempt.'

Allison looks worried, and I can tell she feels it's a bad decision. 'Can I have a look at your Epirb?' she asks. She opens up our Epirb box, inspecting the new 406 system. If the Epirb is activated, it is only a matter of minutes before rescue services are notified, although if you're in the middle of the Atlantic, where we'll be in just a couple of days, it could be a long time before you're picked up.

The transducer area is braced and we nervously head back out to sea. 'I want the bilge pump off,' I say to Adrian as we exit the port, 'and I want you to note down exactly how much water comes in every 15 minutes.' This will allow us to gauge if the damage is getting worse or not. He comes up into the helm a few minutes later looking pleased.

'Just one cup of water in there, which is what we had after the repair anyway.' This is good news, as it means the Splashzone is holding. I lean back in the driver's seat, still anxious about our precarious situation.

A couple of hours later and we're nearing Gibraltar. Shortly we'll be in the Atlantic Ocean, and from there it should be a nice following sea all the way to Barbados. That's what the forecasts are showing at least. Adrian disappears forward for his checks, then comes hurtling back looking pale. 'Pete. You need to have a look at this.' There's urgency to his voice, like we're about to sink.

We scamper forward and, sure enough, the forward section is filling up rapidly. We turn on the bilge pump, and the water level stabilises for a few minutes then gradually starts to recede. It means already the leak has opened up to a size where it almost exceeds the pump's ability to expel water. Clambering down inside the narrow compartment, I feel my way along the damaged zone. The bracing has gone and the transducer plate is now almost free. There are also a number of new soft zones where the foam underneath is waterlogged and crumbling to bits, further compromising hull integrity. 'We need to return to Malaga now,' I say, with finality.

Three hours later and we're back on the dock. Scott has a cunning plan to fix the leak and weakened areas, but it'll take at least 12 hours — and I'm not really convinced it'll hold. A major problem is we were unable to stem the flow of water completely last time, and so we cannot use normal composites in the repair. And now the leaks are much worse, and the damage area has increased.

## If we get the repairs done, they will only be good for flat conditions or a following sea

The whole team sits down and everyone throws in their ideas. Scott and Allison are both really worried but not wanting to say it. Ryan looks tired and dejected, as though he knows it's over. John would like us to continue if safe, because we still have sponsor obligations to meet. Gandhi says he'll go with the flow, and Adrian wants to patch the leak and leave tonight.

'A big problem for us,' I start, 'is we're now into hurricane season. If we get the repairs done, they will only be good for flat conditions or a following sea. If we get into a storm I reckon we'd be buggered. To do a proper repair would take at least three days, and that leaves us no chance of getting the record.' Scott and Allison are nodding in agreement. 'So I think we should call it off.'

There's silence around the group. No one speaks for ages.

'I think it's the right decision,' Allison says finally. I look over at Ryan and he's got a tear rolling down his cheek. *Earthrace* has been our life for years, and in the space of a few hours it's suddenly at an end.

'You know team, we need to remember what we set out to do . . . and that is to promote biodiesel. We've given over 130 TV interviews. We've

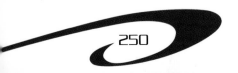

been on NBC, CNN, BBC, PBS, Discovery and The History Channel. There have been countless newspaper and magazine articles. Hell, we even got in *Playboy*.' A wry smile emerges on Ryan's face. 'You may not realise it, but we've connected with millions of people. And while we didn't get the record, we're still a success — and we did try our best, which is all we can do. So forget fixing the leak now. Let's go have a beer and celebrate what we did achieve.'

My mind suddenly drifts off to New Zealand. The worst thing about *Earthrace* has been the enormous strain I've placed on Sharyn and my two girls by being away for so long. At times I felt like just giving it all away and going home. Well, now I can. I grab the sat phone and seconds later I'm talking to my wife, soul mate, best friend and lover. 'Sharyn, I'm coming home.'

There's a long pause on the end of the line. 'I'll have the rum and coke ready for ya.'

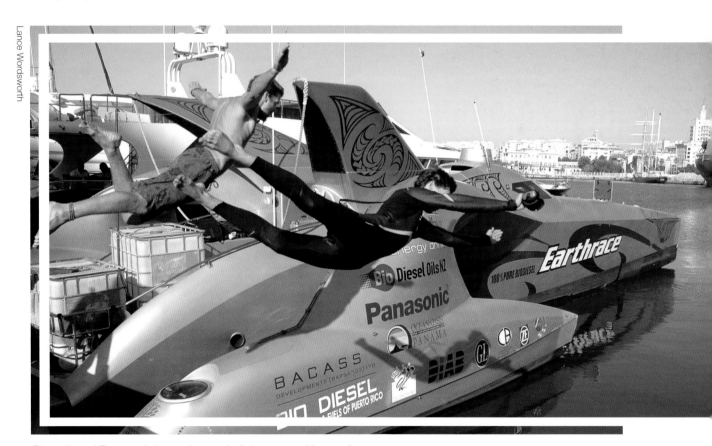

Lance Wordsworth

Ghandi and Ryan celebrate the end of the race with a swim.

# Epilogue

The winter sun warms my cheeks as I sit on our front porch and admire our puka plants. It's amazing how much they've grown since we started Earthrace. It's midday and my day is unfolding like any other over the last month. I get up around 7am and go for a run with Sharyn, drop the kids at school around 8.30, work on my book for a few hours, grab lunch, a few more hours on the book, then pick the girls up. It's been a revelation just chilling out in such a low-stress environment, having some time with the family, and getting my mind and body back in order.

When I first got back, Sharyn and I went for a run and I only made it a couple of kilometres before giving up. Sharyn had this cheeky little smirk on her face suggesting I'd turned into a soft wuss. During the race I never fully appreciated how much it was affecting our bodies and minds. Our fitness just deteriorated, and even now, six weeks after returning, I'm still nowhere near the fitness I had pre-race.

It was several weeks back in New Zealand before I managed to sleep through the night. I'd wake every three or four hours for my turn at driving. There was also this on going nightmare that Ryan and I had in common that kept returning. I've fallen asleep at the wheel and we're running onto rocks. Or something along those lines. I'd jump out of bed groping around desperately for the helm chair and steering wheel hidden somewhere in the darkness of our bedroom. Eventually I'd slide back into bed defeated, or wake up bathed in sweat with the realisation that the same dream continues to haunt me. Time and family though are great healers, and for two weeks now I've slept right through the night.

I look down at the base of our puka plant beside me and Banjo, our pet rabbit, is lying there stretched out like a cat. He's kind of half dog, half cat.

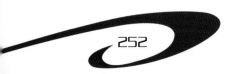

He's a giant Flemish, and about the size of a dog, and he sits there beside me like a faithful friend each day. I reach over and he lifts his head towards me, allowing me to scratch the bit of fur between his ears. A year or so ago I built a fence to keep him in, but he's like the great Houdini, escaping through various nooks and crannies. So he's become the neighbourhood's free-range rabbit, munching on everyone's gardens as he pleases, and returning each morning to keep me company.

I had never really imagined life like this after the race. I'd always thought we'd just get the record, finish our sponsor obligations, and I'd get back to a normal 9 to 5 job. All along it seemed there was something special about Earthrace, as if our team and the boat combined were invincible, and that we were destined to get the record. We had so many challenges thrown at us, and each time we bounced back and overcame them, only to be faced with a new obstacle. And we were always getting ever closer to San Diego with the record time still in sight.

For the moment the boat is up the Baltic Sea running promotions. While I was flying back home, the remaining team members pulled *Earthrace* from the water and repaired the damaged hull and various other bruises and scrapes we'd subjected our amazing boat to. I'd certainly made the right decision to call off the record attempt. The cracks around the transducer only had to work another thirty centimetres forward or back and we'd have been dead in the water.

There is talk of making another record attempt in March 2008. It's funny how the ground crew were keen from day one to do this, while those of us who'd persevered on the boat couldn't think of anything worse. Now though, we're warming to the idea. A German company Deutsche Med has recently taken us under their wing and are keen to be involved in a second go. Cummins Mercruiser and ZF Marine have also offered to support us again. So another attempt is not definite, but it gets more likely by the day.

I'm now getting a constant trickle of emails from obscure naval architects, boat builders or amateurs wanting information on the tri-hull wave-piercing design. Craig Loomes has deservedly picked up a number of jobs designing variations on *Earthrace*, albeit less extreme, and several of these have already been launched. So it seems the design is destined to evolve further and become a small part of naval architecture history.

The National Bank continues to hassle us as if we're dodgy customers. When I turn up at the bank to make a withdrawal, the teller's screen flashes a warning that 'it must be approved by the special administrator' (who threatened us part way into the race). The tellers though all know us by now, and gracefully excuse themselves to make the call, then come back looking pleased that 'yes, in this instance I can withdraw the thousand dollars'. I owe a king's ransom across the Middle East, North America and Europe, but with the National Bank it's now just like a normal mortgage. If I had a good rant they'd likely put things all back to normal, but right now I can't really be bothered. Life is so good that I'm not really fussed. When you've been shot at by the Colombian navy, detained under armed guard at a military base, and survived 12-metre waves, a few hassles at the bank are actually kinda nice . . . and for now our house at least is safe.

Banjo clambers up on my lap. His big paws are on my thigh and he's craning his head up towards my sandwich that I'm holding in the air. He knows if he hassles me enough I'll give him some goodies out of the middle. I pull out the lettuce and hand it over. He settles down munching it in my lap, spreading smears of mayonnaise on my track pants.

My mind wanders back to the amazing dream that was Earthrace. There are many reasons why we made it as far as we did. Firstly, we believed in what we were doing, and for that you're prepared to sacrifice a lot. Secondly, there was an army of volunteers and supporters as well as ground crews who similarly believed in what Earthrace stands for, and who worked tirelessly on our behalf.

Thirdly, many people gave the performance of their lives to Earthrace. The project was a brutal challenge that demanded so much time, energy and resources from a dedicated band of people, and many of them were simply outstanding in what they delivered.

Finally, we had the support of an array of sponsors, especially Cummins Mercruiser and ZF Marine who called on their global network to assist us almost anywhere in the world. I remember the three Cummins technicians in India who worked non-stop for almost a day, in the darkest and tiniest engine bay, and in 45°C heat. When they walked out they almost collapsed from exhaustion.

In the end, though, this wasn't enough to get the record, and there are several reasons why. Peter Blake, in his first attempt to claim the Jules Verne Trophy, hit something in the water and ended up calling the attempt off. He said to the media afterwards, 'To get around the globe in record time, you need a little bit of luck along the way'. Well, the same certainly applied to us, and I'm not sure we had much luck go our way. When I sit back and consider the specifics, though, on why we didn't get the record, most of the things were well within our control.

We left it too late to install the new carbon propellers, and as a result we never found out they were deficient until the record attempt had started. We should have had these running months earlier for thorough sea trials. Next came the collision near Guatemala. While the Guatemalan fishermen were asleep, and with no solid white light, and these are major contributors to the accident, I still believe that if Anthony had been right on top of things, he'd have picked them up on radar. In addition to the lost time we incurred in Guatemala, and then in San Diego effecting repairs, we were now pushed into monsoon and hurricane season, the adverse weather of which was our final undoing.

We also lost a week in Palau waiting on a spare piston to arrive. We originally intended to have a spare with us, and when it never arrived with our other parts in Charleston, we should have followed up and ensured we got it before the race started.

Our logistical support in India was very poor, costing us many days waiting for fuel that then turned out to be dodgy. The engine mounts were also under-designed, although in the end this never really cost us any time, just stress. The final hull failure that stopped the attempt is probably the one thing outside our control. The designers had intended the transducer be installed using a particular method, but this information was not relayed to the boat builders. Calibre Boats used a technique typical of what they use on other boats, but this was not up to the continued poundings *Earthrace* was subjected to. In fairness, though, it is unbelievable that there haven't been other structural issues with *Earthrace*. It has weathered brutal and enormous seas in so many storms, and it is amazing that, after all that, we had but a single structural failure.

Craig Loomes, Calibre Boats and Germansche Lloyd I believe were outstanding in delivering us an amazing boat. The transducer plate failure was just the final element in our not getting the record, but if we'd been on top of all the other things I've mentioned, we'd have been able to simply effect repairs in Malaga and continue on to get the record anyway. So in the end we let ourselves down in a few key areas, and that is why we didn't get the record. We did our best, though, and that's all we can do . . . but in the end it wasn't good enough.

The big regret I have with Earthrace remains the accident in Guatemala; firstly, that it happened at all and, secondly, my actions immediately following the accident. If I had swum over to Pajarito first, instead of rescuing Gonzalez, we'd have brought all three men aboard. With the qualified doctor and good first-aid supplies at our disposal, we'd have had a good chance of saving all three fishermen rather than just the two. I made the wrong decision at the time and it is something I'll have to live with. Pajarito's family of course bear a much heavier burden than I. The only positive was that our actions and medical treatment of Gonzalez saved his life, but it is little consolation to Pajarito's family.

I remember Ryan coming into my room the morning after we'd called off the race. He was heading back to New Zealand to start editing the TV series. He'd given up over two years of his life to *Earthrace*, and had remained a staunch and loyal supporter throughout. The strange thing is I never quite knew what to say. In the end it was just a quick 'See ya later and thanks', and suddenly he was gone. It felt like I'd just lost a friend. The team then seemed somehow empty without him.

But the cool thing with the Earthrace project is that it is bigger than just a few team members or a boat. It is an army of people who all believe we can make a small difference with our actions, and we'll continue to do so.

A final thank you to all who have supported us on this most amazing adventure. I've always believed anyone who got to crew on *Earthrace* was privileged, because it was only through the efforts of many hundreds of people and sponsors who went before them that *Earthrace* exists at all. Well I've been at the centre of this journey, and in the most privileged position of all. To have people you don't even know, or meet briefly on a dock, who then front up and help, donate or sponsor is a humbling experience indeed, and I'm extremely grateful to have been in such an enviable position. So thank you again for making such an incredible project possible. Like many others on *Earthrace*, this has enabled me to live the dream and follow something I believe in, and we've hopefully made a positive contribution in the process.

### Lessons I have learned from Earthrace

'I'd like you to talk about what lessons you've learned from Earthrace, especially those that contributed to your success.' That was what Ross Brown, the Principal of Napier Boys High School, had said to me before I talked to their assembly in 2006. It wasn't something I'd really thought about much, and on the day I was less than eloquent in delivering my thoughts. Since then, though, I've gradually put together a few of the key things I've learned. I guess many of you will think they're obvious, but someone out there might find them helpful.

### Stand up for what you believe in

If you believe in something then stand up for it. Be proactive and believe that what you do matters, and that you can make a difference. Also let people know your feelings and opinions, and speak from the heart. Why exactly do you care? If others understand your reasoning, maybe they'll take a similar view.

### Have faith

There were many times when Earthrace seemed doomed, but I always had faith that one way or another, we would pull it off. I believed in the message, the team and the boat, and I knew that we would make a positive contribution with what we were doing. Sometimes, though, it felt like Sharyn and I were the only ones who could see this. I remember meeting a lady at Tourism New Zealand and she said to me, 'It's just a boat. Why would anyone be interested in it?' Well soon we'll be celebrating the 100,000th person through *Earthrace*. In the end people were interested, but early on there were only a few of us who could see it.

### Give things a go

I have always had a strong sense of wanting to try things. I had not raced a boat before, but that didn't stop me from attempting the speed record. I'd never raised a cent of sponsorship before, but that didn't stop me from knocking on corporate doors. Some might say poorly, of course, but we did raise enough to get *Earthrace* launched and around the globe. I had never taken a boat out of sight of land before, and yet I skippered *Earthrace* across the Pacific Ocean. Right now I'm writing my first book. Just get out there and do it. You should not be afraid of failure, but rather of not doing anything at all. This follows a great Kiwi tradition of people who just get out there and do things.

*If at first you don't succeed, try another approach*

When we first started Earthrace, we had very clear ideas on what we wanted to achieve, and how we would go about getting there. However, many of our original ideas and plans just didn't work out. At times it felt like we were bashing our heads against a brick wall. So we started trying new methods or ideas, and if they worked, we moved on, and if they didn't, we'd try something else. Don't just keep trying the same things if they continue to fail. Think laterally and work around the problem.

*Surround yourself with good people*

One of the great things with Earthrace is that it attracted so many people willing to help us — a fantastic pool of talent that we could draw on. Many of these people had skills or experience that made up for my lack of them. Over a four-year period we had hundreds and hundreds of people donate their time to us, in one form or other. For some it might just be a few hours and for others, like Ryan, years of their life. From this large pool, we could cherry pick really capable people and get them to remain on the team for sustained periods. Not all of course are in a position to give up weeks, months or years of their lives, but some are. And sometimes you cannot get the outstanding people you might want, but always aim for it at least. Related to this is ensuring your team has integrity, and getting rid of any who don't.

*Do the best with what you've got*

This developed as our philosophy early on. Right through Earthrace we remained under-resourced for what we were trying to achieve, so we just did our best with what we had. In many cases we had to be creative or flexible in how we did things, and sometimes it wasn't as pretty as we'd have liked. It is also a case of prioritising the most important things leading to your goals, and ensuring those are met, then working down the order.

*Value and nurture your friends and family*

One of our great strengths has been our ability to gather in friends and family to help the cause. Examples are old mates from school who loaned me tens of thousands of dollars at crucial times. There were many people who selflessly turned up at the yard, weekend after weekend, to sand the hull or work during promotions. We were given houses around the country and overseas for the crew to stay in. When things got financially desperate for Sharyn during the race, many family members and friends would turn up at our house with food parcels or just to help out. Nurturing friends is especially relevant to kids. School friends are the best mates you'll probably ever have, mostly because you share such an array of fantastic experiences with them that vary as you go through life. These people are also the most likely to help you later on in life. So make sure you look after them.

Kia Kaha.

# *Earthrace* specifications

| | |
|---|---|
| Hull: | Wave-piercing trimaran |
| Designer: | Craig Loomes Design |
| Length: | 24 metres (78 feet) |
| Beam: | 8 metres (26 feet) |
| Draft: | 1.3 metres (4 feet) |
| Range: | 2000–5000 nautical miles (3500–9000 kilometres depending on speed) |
| Maximum speed: | 40 knots (75 km/h), depending on fuel load and propellers |
| Fuel: | B100 Biodiesel (100%) |
| Fuel capacity: | 14,000 litres (3500 gallons) |
| Dry weight: | 14 tonnes |
| Construction: | Carbon, Kevlar composites |
| Crew: | 4 |
| Beds: | 6 |
| Engines: | 2 x 350 kilowatt (540 horsepower) Cummins Mercruiser QS 540 |
| Gearboxes: | ZF 305A (single speed) |
| Air intakes: | Top of wings to remain above waves while piercing |
| Windscreen: | 17 millimetres (¾ inch) laminated toughened glass |

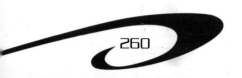